McGRAW·HILL

HEALTH

TEACHER'S BLACKLINE MASTERS • GRADE 5

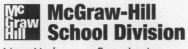

**McGraw-Hill
School Division**

New York   Farmington

McGraw-Hill School Division

A Division of The McGraw-Hill Companies

Copyright © 1999 McGraw-Hill School Division, a Division of the Educational
and Professional Publishing Group of The McGraw-Hill Companies, Inc.

McGraw-Hill School Division
1221 Avenue of the Americas
New York, New York 10020

Printed in the United States of America
ISBN 0-02-276879-3 / 5
1 2 3 4 5 6 7 8 9 045 03 02 01 00 99 98 97

Contents

Name: _____ Date: _____

Dear Parent or Guardian,

We are about to start **Chapter 1, Personal Health**, in which we will explore this Big Idea:

> Staying in good health involves knowing how to take care of yourself and going to the right people when you need help.

Your child will be learning about

- the importance of developing good personal health care habits
- the proper care of teeth and gums
- the care of eyes and ears
- protecting and caring for skin, hair, and nails

Help your child fill out the checklist below. Talk about how practicing ideas from the checklist can help your family keep fit and feel better.

Personal Health Family Checklist

☐ Our family understands that staying healthy means making healthful choices about physical, emotional and intellectual, and social health.

☐ We each follow a daily grooming routine and get plenty of rest and sleep.

☐ We get regular physical checkups.

☐ We brush and floss our teeth daily and get regular dental checkups.

☐ Children and adults protect their eyes by wearing safety goggles and sunglasses when necessary.

☐ We know that loud noises can cause hearing loss.

☐ Children and adults wear sunscreen with a SPF of at least 15.

☐ We have the necessary tools and products for the proper care of our teeth, skin, hair, and nails.

If you are interested in learning more about personal health, a good resource is: *Fit for Life* **(Franklin Watts, 1996)**.

McGraw-Hill School Division

Name: _____ Date: _____

WHAT IS HEALTH?

Complete each sentence with a word from the box. You may use a word more than once.

| physical | emotional | intellectual | social |

1. Eating well and being physically active is taking care of your

   _____health.

2. You maintain your _____ health when you make and keep

   friends.

3. Working in groups and getting along with others can improve your

   _____ health.

4. Expressing your feelings helps maintain your _____ health.

5. Learning new things is part of good _____ health.

6. Respecting yourself is part of good _____ health.

Answer each question with complete sentences.

7. What are the three parts of health?

   _____

8. Why can't you control every aspect of your health?

   _____

9. What are two signs that a person is emotionally and intellectually
   healthy?

   _____

10. What would you do before following any advice about your health?

    _____

    _____

Name: _____   Date: _____

WHAT IS HEALTH?

Match the word or words in Column A with the description in Column B.
Write the correct letter in the blank.

Column A

___ **1.** emotional and intellectual health

___ **2.** healthful

___ **3.** physical health

___ **4.** risk

___ **5.** social health

Column B

A. involves relationships with other people

B. related to your mind and feelings

C. good for your health

D. deals with the condition of your body

E. possibility of loss or harm

Answer each question in complete sentences.

6. What are the three parts of health?

_____

7. What are three factors that affect your health?

_____

8. How can the people you know help you stay healthy?

_____

9. In what two ways could you avoid risk to your physical health?

_____

10. What is a healthful choice you can make that would help you stay well?

_____

Name: _____ Date: _____

PERSONAL HEALTH CARE

Write True or False for each statement. If the statement is false, change the underlined word or phrase to make it true.

_____ 1. Responsibility for your health belongs mostly to your family.

_____ 2. When you look neat and smell fresh, you improve your emotional and social health.

_____ 3. During stage 1 of sleep, your muscles slowly relax.

_____ 4. Body temperature and blood pressure rise during stage 3 of sleep.

_____ 5. Medical and dental records can provide useful information about your medical history.

Write the word or phrase from the box that best completes each sentence.

| once a year   twice a year   10–11 hours |
| 90 minutes   5–15 minutes |

6. For the health of your teeth, you should have a dental checkup at least

_____ .

7. To be well rested, most young people need about _____ of

sleep a day.

8. During a night's sleep, each REM period lasts about _____.

9. To maintain your health, it is a good idea to have a medical checkup at least

_____.

10. You enter the REM stage about _____ after you fall asleep.

Name: _____ Date: _____

PERSONAL HEALTH CARE

Write the word or phrase that best completes each sentence.

1. The care of one's appearance is _____.

2. The way you carry your body is your _____.

3. The condition of being clean is called _____.

4. The quick jerking of the eye during the dream stage of sleep is called

   _____.

Answer each question with complete sentences.

5. What are two ways in which good grooming keeps you healthy?

   _____

   _____

6. What can a person's posture tell you about that person?

   _____

7. How does sleep affect personal health?

   _____

8. Why is it important to get regular medical checkups?

   _____

9. What does a doctor usually do during a medical checkup?

   _____

   _____

10. Why is it important to go to the dentist regularly?

   _____

   _____

Name: _____   Date: _____

ORAL HEALTH

Underline the phrase that best completes each sentence.

1. By the time you have reached the age of 21, you will probably have (32, 24) teeth.

2. Your teeth play an important part in the (digestive, breathing) process.

3. To bite off a piece of celery for a snack, you most likely use your (molars, incisors).

4. The white, protective outer layer of a tooth is the (crown, enamel).

5. It's best to floss (when food gets stuck between your teeth, at least once a day).

6. The (gum, pulp) surrounds each tooth and helps keep it in place.

7. (Pyorrhea, Caries) is a kind of tooth decay that produces small holes in the teeth.

8. An orthodontist might use (braces, root canal therapy) to correct malocclusion.

Answer each question with complete sentences.

9. What is the difference between the root and the crown of a tooth?

_____

_____

10. Why would a dentist use a cap or a bridge to repair teeth?

_____

_____

_____

Name: _____ Date: _____

ORAL HEALTH

Complete the definition of each word.

1. Enamel is _____

2. Plaque is _____

3. Gingivitis is _____

4. Tartar is _____

5. Fluoride is _____

Answer each question in complete sentences.

6. How do teeth affect your appearance?

_____

_____

7. Where is the root of a tooth located?

_____

8. What are two ways in which bacteria can cause tooth or gum problems?

_____

_____

9. What can happen if you let plaque build up on your teeth?

_____

_____

10. What can you do to take care of your teeth and gums?

_____

_____

Name: _____   Date: _____

EYE CARE

Complete each sentence with a word or words from the box.

iris	cone cells	conjunctiva
ophthalmologist	optic nerve	rod cells

1. The colored portion of the eye that controls the amount of light coming in is the _____.

2. The color of light is sensed by _____.

3. The brightness of light is sensed by _____.

4. The _____ connects your eye to your brain.

5. The sensitive lining of the eyelid is the _____.

6. An _____ examines eyes and can prescribe medicine, glasses, contact lenses, or surgery.

Match the word or words in Column A with the description in Column B. Write the correct letter in the blank.

Column A

_____ 7. astigmatism

_____ 8. conjunctivitis

_____ 9. farsightedness

_____ 10. nearsightedness

Column B

A. pink eye that results when eyelid lining becomes infected

B. lengthening of eyeball makes it difficult to focus on distant objects

C. blurred vision caused by irregularly shaped cornea or lens

D. shortening of eyeball makes it difficult to focus on nearby objects

McGraw-Hill School Division

Name: _____   Date: _____

EYE CARE

Write the word that will best complete each sentence.

1. The covering that protects the front of the eye is the _____.

2. The curved, clear part of the eye behind the pupil is the _____.

3. The lining along the back of the eyeball is the _____.

4. The opening that lets light enter the eye is the _____.

5. Doctors who treat eye diseases and disorders are _____.

Answer each question with complete sentences.

6. How do tears protect your eyes?

_____

7. What can you do to protect your eyes from damage?

_____

_____

_____

Write the word or phrase from the box that best completes each sentence.

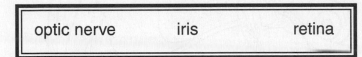

| optic nerve | iris | retina |

8. Light enters the eye through the pupil at the center of the
_____.

9. The lens focuses and projects the image on the _____,
where the image is upside down.

10. Rod and cone cells transform light rays into nerve impulses that travel
along the _____ to the brain.

Name: _____   Date: _____

EAR CARE

Write True or False for each statement. If false, change the underlined word or phrase to make it true.

_____ **1.** Three bones in the middle ear are the hammer, anvil, and <u>cochlea</u>.

_____ **2.** The outer part of the ear canal is lined with fine hairs and <u>wax-producing glands</u>.

_____ **3.** The <u>auricle</u> separates the outer ear from the middle ear.

_____ **4.** An audiologist <u>prescribes medicine for ear infections</u>.

_____ **5.** Exposure to <u>very loud noise</u> can cause permanent hearing loss.

Choose a word or phrase from the box to label each part of the diagram.

auditory nerve   cochlea   ear canal   eardrum   sound waves

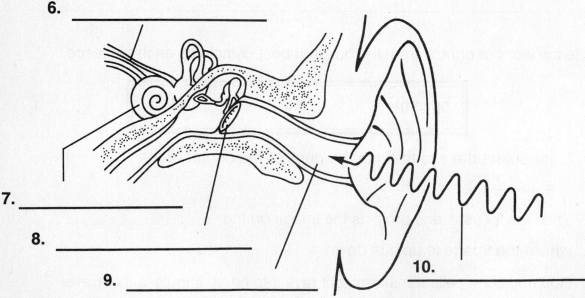

6. _____

7. _____

8. _____

9. _____

10. _____

Name: _____   Date: _____

EAR CARE

Write the word that will best complete each sentence.

1. The funnel-shaped outer part of the ear is the _____.

2. The thin tissue in the ear that vibrates with sound is the _____.

3. A unit used to measure the loudness of a sound is a _____.

4. A person who tests hearing is an _____.

5. Tiny microphones that help conduct sound are _____.

6. Use the letters **a**, **b**, **c**, **d**, and **e** to order the steps that explain how you hear.

_____ Messages travel along the auditory nerve to the brain.

_____ The eardrum vibrates and bones in the middle ear strengthen the vibrations.

_____ The brain senses sound and you respond.

_____ Sound waves enter the outer ear and travel through the ear canal.

_____ Vibrations produce waves in the inner ear.

Answer each question with complete sentences.

7. What happens if anything goes wrong with the way the ear works?

_____

8. How do wax-producing glands in the ear canal protect your ears?

_____

9. How can exposure to very loud sounds cause hearing loss?

_____

10. What rules should you follow to take care of your ears?

_____

_____

Name: _____ Date: _____

SKIN, HAIR, AND NAIL CARE

Underline the phrase that best completes each sentence.

1. (Cells, Pores) are the smallest living parts of the body.

2. Hair and nails are a thickened form of (fatty tissue, epidermis).

3. (Acne, Athlete's foot) is a skin infection caused by a fungus.

4. The higher the SPF, the more protection you have against (harmful sun rays, insect bites).

5. Sharing combs or brushes is not a good idea because it spreads (head lice, dandruff).

6. The special skin that surrounds the nails of your fingers and toes is called the (follicle, cuticle).

Answer each question with complete sentences.

7. What are pimples and what produces them?

   _____

   _____

8. How should sunscreen be used?

   _____

   _____

   _____

9. What do fingernails do?

   _____

10. What are three tools you can use to care for your nails?

    _____

Grade 5, Chapter 1, Lesson 6

Name: _____   Date: _____

SKIN, HAIR, AND NAIL CARE

Match the word or words in Column A with the description in Column B.
Write the correct letter in the blank.

Column A

_____ 1. epidermis

_____ 2. follicle

_____ 3. melanin

_____ 4. pore

_____ 5. sunscreen

Column B

A. a small hole, or sac, in the skin that holds a hair root

B. a tiny opening in the skin's surface

C. a cream or lotion that helps protect skin from the harmful rays of the sun

D. the protective outer layer of skin

E. a dark pigment in skin

Answer each question in complete sentences.

6. What are two functions of the skin?

_____

7. What is the difference between the epidermis and the dermis?

_____

_____

_____

8. How do sweat glands in skin help control body temperature?

_____

9. What three things could happen if you don't wash your skin regularly?

_____

_____

10. Why should you brush and comb your hair every day?

_____

Name: _____   Date: _____

PERSONAL HEALTH

Write the word from the box that best completes each sentence.

cornea	eardrum	enamel
epidermis	follicle	grooming
plaque	posture	retina	risk

1. The hard, white, protective outer layer of a tooth is _____ .

2. The care of one's appearance is _____ .

3. The lining along the back of the eyeball is the _____ .

4. A possibility of loss or harm is _____ .

5. The sticky film containing germs that forms on teeth is _____ .

6. The clear outer covering that protects the front of the eye is the

    _____ .

7. The protective outer layer of skin is the _____ .

8. The thin tissue in the ear that vibrates with sound is the _____ .

9. The way you carry your body is _____ .

10. A hole, or sac, in the dermis that holds a hair root is a _____ .

Write <u>True</u> or <u>False</u> for each statement. If false, change the underlined word or phrase to make it true.

_____ 11. <u>Astigmatism</u> is treated by wearing glasses with corrective lenses.

_____ 12. The most important job for your teeth is to help you <u>speak</u>.

_____ 13. The nerves in your skin allow you to <u>feel heat, cold, pressure, and pain.</u>

Name: _____   Date: _____

PERSONAL HEALTH

_____ 14. Being able to think clearly and solve problems is an example of <u>emotional and intellectual health</u>.

_____ 15. The <u>optic nerve</u> passes messages from the inner ear to the brain.

_____ 16. During the REM stage of sleep, the body twitches, eyes move, and <u>chewing</u> takes place.

Answer each question with complete sentences.

17. What are head lice and what happens if you get them?

_____

_____

18. How does eating properly affect your oral health?

_____

_____

19. What are two signs that a person is socially healthy?

_____

_____

20. Why shouldn't you use swabs or pointed objects inside your ear?

_____

_____

Extra Credit: On a separate piece of paper, write a paragraph describing a program for improving or maintaining personal health.

McGraw-Hill School Division

Name: _____   Date: _____

Dear Parent or Guardian,

We are about to start **Chapter 2, Growth and Development**, in which we will explore this Big Idea:

> As you go through the stages of life, your body works in many ways that help you grow and develop. By taking good care of your body, you will help keep it functioning well.

Your child will be learning about

- the stages of human development
- how good health practices can affect development
- the parts and functions of the skeletal and muscular systems
- the roles of the circulatory and respiratory systems
- the processes of digestion and excretion
- the roles of the nervous and endocrine systems

Help your child fill out the checklist below. Talk about how practicing ideas from the checklist can help your family members keep their bodies functioning well.

**Growth and Development
Family Checklist**

☐ Our family members are aware that people grow and change throughout their lives.

☐ We recognize the physical and emotional changes that characterize adolescence.

☐ We understand that the proper functioning of our body systems depends on healthy choices we make for ourselves.

☐ We get the proper amount of rest.

☐ We know that a balanced diet, regular physical activity, and good habits contribute to our healthy growth and development.

☐ Family members wear and use appropriate safety equipment to prevent injuries to the spine and brain.

☐ For a healthy heart and lungs, we avoid smoking.

If you are interested in learning more about growth and development, a good resource is: Laura Nathanson's **The Portable Pediatrician's Guide to Kids**, (HarperPerennial, 1996).

Name: _____   Date: _____

STAGES OF LIFE

Write the word or phrase from the box that best completes each sentence.

| adolescence   childhood   environment   health practices   traits |

1. During _____ you learn many good health habits, such as keeping clean, eating well, and brushing your teeth.

2. A period of rapid growth is very common during _____.

3. Many of your characteristics, or _____, were inherited from your parents.

4. The air you breathe is part of your _____.

5. Eating a balanced diet and getting plenty of rest are good _____.

Write True or False for each statement. If false, change the underlined word or phrase to make it true.

_____ 6. It is very unusual for a growth spurt to happen during a person's adolescence.

_____ 7. As an adolescent, the number and difficulty of your tasks at home and at school will probably increase.

_____ 8. Both heredity and environment play a part in your growth and development.

_____ 9. You did not choose your inherited traits.

_____ 10. Infancy is a time of slow growth and development.

Name: _____   Date: _____

STAGES OF LIFE

Match the word in Column A with the description in Column B.
Write the correct letter in the blank.

Column A

_____ 1. adolescence

_____ 2. environment

_____ 3. heredity

_____ 4. growth spurt

_____ 5. puberty

Column B

A. passing of traits from parents to children

B. stage of life between childhood and adulthood

C. the stage when an adolescent begins to take on the physical characteristics of an adult

D. your surroundings

E. a period of rapid growth that is very common during adolescence

Answer each question in complete sentences.

6. What are four stages of development that people go through?

_____

7. During what stage of development does puberty occur?

_____

8. What are some inherited traits?

_____

_____

9. What are some parts of your environment?

_____

_____

10. Why is following safety rules a good health habit?

_____

Name: _____ Date: _____

THE BODY—FROM CELLS TO SYSTEMS

Write the word or phrase from the box that matches each picture.

cell	body system	organ

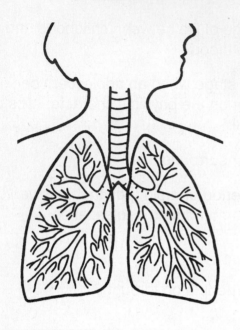

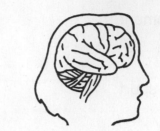

2. _____

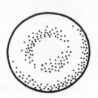

1. _____   3. _____

Underline the phrase that best completes each sentence.

4. The growth and division of cells occurs at a (rapid, slow) rate.

5. A basic job of cells is to take in (carbon dioxide, oxygen).

6. (Nerve cells, skin cells) bring messages from your eyes to your brain.

7. The brain is made up largely of (muscle, nerve) tissue.

8. A (tissue, organ) is a group of similar cells that work together to do a job.

9. The stomach and intestines are part of the (skeletal, digestive) body system.

10. (Cells, Hearts) are the basic structural units of living things.

Name: _____   Date: _____

THE BODY—FROM CELLS TO SYSTEMS

Match the word or words in Column A with the description in Column B.
Write the correct letter in the blank.

Column A

_____ 1. body system

_____ 2. cell

_____ 3. organ

_____ 4. tissue

Column B

A. the basic structural unit of life

B. a group of similar cells that work together to do a certain job

C. a group of organs that work together to perform a particular job for the body

D. a group of tissues that has a specific form and function

Answer each question in complete sentences.

5. What are the four basic jobs of cells?

_____

_____

6. How does cell reproduction allow your body to grow and develop?

_____

7. What are three organs in your digestive system?

_____

8. What is the job of nerve cells?

_____

9. Your heart is mostly made up of which kind of tissue?

_____

10. For what job is the muscular system needed?

_____

Name: _____   Date: _____

YOUR BONES AND MUSCLES

Write the word or phrase from the box that matches each pictured body part.

```
contracted muscle    hinge joint    relaxed muscle    tendon
```

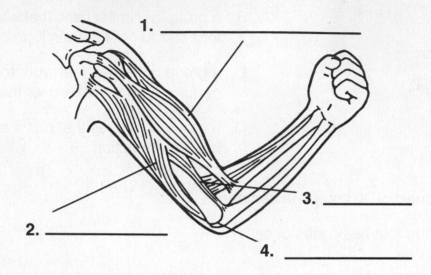

1. _____

2. _____

3. _____

4. _____

Underline the phrase that best completes each sentence.

5. The human body contains about (100, 200) bones.

6. The bones of the body support your weight, enable you to move, and protect your (internal organs, skin).

7. Immovable joints are found in the (elbow, skull).

8. The ends of some bones are protected by flexible tissue called (cartilage, ligaments).

9. Heart muscle is an example of (involuntary muscle, voluntary muscle).

10. Special care for sprains is called "RICE", which is the abbreviation for Rest, Ice, Compression, and (Elevation, Exercise).

Name: _____   Date: _____

YOUR BONES AND MUSCLES

Write the word that will best complete each sentence.

1. Flexible tissue that covers and protects the ends of some bones is _____.

2. Muscles that you can control are called _____.

3. Strong cords of tissue that connect muscles to bones are _____.

4. Strong bands of tissue that hold bones together at a joint are _____.

5. A place where two bones meet is a _____.

Answer each question in complete sentences.

6. What are the three jobs that your skeletal system does?

   _____

   _____

7. How do your bones get longer as you grow?

   _____

8. How do voluntary and involuntary muscles differ in the way they function?

   _____

   _____

9. How do pairs of skeletal muscles work together?

   _____

10. How can you take care of a sprain by RICE?

    _____

    _____

McGraw-Hill School Division

Name: _____ Date: _____

YOUR HEART AND LUNGS

Write True or False for each statement. If false, change the underlined word or phrase to make it true.

_____ **1.** The circulatory system <u>gets rid of</u> oxygen, food, and other materials throughout the body.

_____ **2.** The circulatory system is made up of the heart, <u>lungs</u>, and blood.

_____ **3.** <u>Platelets</u> are cell fragments that help the blood to clot.

_____ **4.** <u>White</u> blood cells carry oxygen throughout the body.

_____ **5.** Smoking is <u>good</u> for the respiratory system.

_____ **6.** The movement of air into and out of your lungs is controlled by the <u>diaphragm</u>.

Write the word or phrase from the box that matches each pictured part.

artery	capillaries	heart	vein

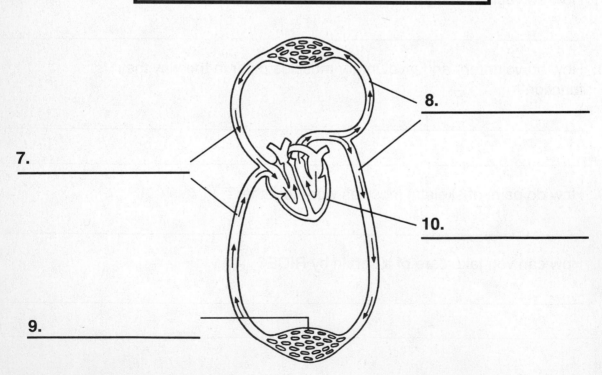

8. _____

7. _____

10. _____

9. _____

Name: _____ Date: _____

YOUR HEART AND LUNGS

Match the word in Column A with the description in Column B.
Write the correct letter in the blank.

Column A

_____ 1. alveoli

_____ 2. arteries

_____ 3. capillaries

_____ 4. platelets

_____ 5. veins

Column B

A. blood vessels that carry blood away from the heart

B. cell fragments that help blood to clot

C. tiny air sacs in the lung

D. blood vessels, through which materials are exchanged between blood and body cells

E. blood vessels that carry blood toward the heart

Answer each question in complete sentences.

6. What are the three parts of the circulatory system?

   _____

7. What is the function of arteries?

   _____

8. In what two ways do capillaries help body cells to function?

   _____

   _____

9. How does oxygen in the lungs get into the circulatory system?

   _____

   _____

10. What is one way of caring for your respiratory system?

   _____

   _____

McGraw-Hill School Division

Name: _____ Date: _____

THE DIGESTIVE AND EXCRETORY SYSTEMS

Circle the letter of the best answer.

1. The most important job of the digestive system is to
   a. get food and oxygen to your cells
   b. change food into a form that cells can use
   c. get rid of wastes

2. When you swallow food, it enters a tube called the
   a. esophagus   b. intestine   c. pancreas

3. Digestive juices that help break down food are found in your
   a. lungs   b. heart and pancreas   c. stomach and small intestine

4. A good way to take care of your digestive system is to eat food with a lot of
   a. fiber   b. fat   c. water

5. A substance produced by your liver to aid digestion is
   a. bile   b. villi   c. saliva

6. Undigested food passes into the
   a. bloodstream   b. capillaries   c. large intestine

Underline the phrase that best completes each sentence.

7. Digestion first begins in the (mouth, stomach).

8. Villi are tiny finger-like projections that line the (small intestine, stomach).

9. Tiny filters in the kidneys help to remove (wastes, oxygen) from the blood.

10. Organs of the excretory system are the kidneys and (liver, skin).

Name: _____   Date: _____

THE DIGESTIVE AND EXCRETORY SYSTEMS

Write the word that will best complete each sentence.

1. A liquid that is produced in the liver to help break down food is

    _____.

2. Finger-like projections along the inside of the small intestine that absorb

    digested food are _____.

3. The body's process for getting rid of wastes is called _____.

4. The largest organ in the body is the _____.

5. Foods with a lot of _____ help to keep food moving through

    the digestive system.

Answer each question in complete sentences.

6. What happens to food in your stomach?

    _____

7. How do digested food particles get into the bloodstream from the
    small intestine?

    _____

    _____

    _____

8. What is one way of taking care of your digestive sysem?

    _____

    _____

9. What is the function of kidneys in the excretory system?

    _____

10. How do sweat glands help in the excretory process?

    _____

Name: _____ Date: _____

THE NERVOUS AND ENDOCRINE SYSTEMS

Write True or False for each statement. If false, change the underlined word or phrase to make it true.

_____ 1. The nervous system is made up of your brain, spinal cord, and nerves.

_____ 2. Sensory neurons relay messages to the brain.

_____ 3. The cerebrum controls the muscle coordination and balance.

_____ 4. The deepening of boys' voices at puberty is an example of a secondary sex characteristic.

_____ 5. The endocrine system controls the body with chemical messengers called neurons.

_____ 6. The pituitary gland controls the growth of bones and muscles as well as the action of other glands of the endocrine system.

Write the word or phrase from the box that best completes each sentence.

cerebrum   motor neurons   medulla   puberty

7. Nerves that relay messages to muscles are called _____.

8. The part of the brain that takes up about two thirds of it is the _____.

9. The part of the brain that controls involuntary acts, such as breathing, is the _____.

10. The pituitary gland sends out a hormone that triggers a growth spurt during _____.

Name: _____   Date: _____

THE NERVOUS AND ENDOCRINE SYSTEMS

Match the word or words in Column A with the description in Column B.
Write the correct letter in the blank.

Column A

_____ 1. cerebellum

_____ 2. cerebrum

_____ 3. hormones

_____ 4. medulla

_____ 5. neurons

Column B

A. chemicals made by the body that control growth and many other body processes

B. nerve cells

C. largest part of the brain; controls speech, thought, and senses

D. part of the brain that controls involuntary acts, such as breathing and heart rate

E. part of the brain that controls balance

Answer each question in complete sentences.

6. What are the three parts of your nervous system?

_____

7. Where are two places that you will find sensory neurons in the body?

_____

8. How does the nervous system help you start a race when the starting whistle sounds?

_____

_____

_____

9. Name four important glands in your body.

_____

10. What part does the pituitary gland play in puberty?

_____

_____

Name: _____   Date: _____

GROWTH AND DEVELOPMENT

Write the word or phrase from the box that best completes each sentence.

adolescence	alveoli	arteries	body system	cartilage
hormones	joint	organ	puberty	villi

1. The stage of life between childhood and adulthood is _____.

2. The stage when an adolescent begins to take on the physical characteristics of an adult is _____.

3. Tiny air sacs in the lungs are _____.

4. A group of tissues that has a specific form and function is an _____.

5. A group of organs that work together to perform a particular job for the body is a _____.

6. A place where two bones meet is a _____.

7. Flexible tissue that covers and protects the ends of some bones is _____.

8. Blood vessels that carry blood away from the heart are _____.

9. Finger-like projections along the inside of the small intestine that absorb food are _____.

10. Chemicals made by your body that control growth and many other body processes are _____.

Circle the letter of the best answer.

11. The kind of stimulus your nose is sensitive to is

   a. light   **b.** odor   **c.** pressure

McGraw-Hill School Division

Name: _____ Date: _____

GROWTH AND DEVELOPMENT

12. Absorption of digested food takes place in the

    a. esophagus   **b.** mouth   **c.** small intestine

13. An injury to the medulla may affect your

    a. speech   **b.** breathing   **c.** vision

14. A growth spurt is common during

    a. adolescence   **b.** digestion   **c.** exercise

15. The fact that you have brown eyes is due to your

    a. endocrine   **b.** heredity   **c.** environment

Answer each question in complete sentences.

16. How does the endocrine system control the body?

_____

_____

17. What are the names and functions of the three parts of the blood?

_____

_____

Write True or False for each statement. If false, change the underlined word or phrase to make it true.

_____ **18.** The thyroid gland is located in your neck.

_____ **19.** Stimuli are changes in your environment.

_____ **20.** It is natural for different people to develop at the same rate during adolescence.

Extra Credit: On a separate piece of paper, write a paragraph that explains why an injury to a nerve in the spine is often more serious than an injury to a bone in the leg.

McGraw-Hill School Division

Name: _____   Date: _____

Dear Parent or Guardian,

We are about to start **Chapter 3, Emotional and Intellectual Health**, in which we will explore this Big Idea:

> When you are emotionally and intellectually healthy, you feel good about yourself, get along with others, and deal with stress in a healthful way.

Your child will be learning about

- how self-concept is related to self-esteem
- behaviors that build self-esteem
- emotions and healthful ways to express them
- healthful and harmful stress and ways to manage stress

Help your child fill out the checklist below. Talk about how practicing ideas from the checklist can help your family stay emotionally and intellectually healthy.

Emotional and Intellectual Health
Family Checklist

☐ Our family behaves in ways that build self-esteem, including accepting our strengths and improving our weaknesses.

☐ We admit to and learn from our mistakes, and treat others with respect and courtesy.

☐ Children and adults avoid risk behaviors.

☐ We know that expressing our emotions in healthful ways is part of maintaining our emotional and intellectual health.

☐ When there is conflict, we avoid violence by calming down, communicating, and apologizing when necessary. We seek help when we can't find a resolution.

☐ We are aware that stress can be healthful or harmful.

☐ We practice ways of managing stress and know how to make responsible decisions.

If you are interested in learning more about emotional and intellectual health, some good resources are: *Coping Through Self-Esteem* (**Rosen Publishing Group, 1993**) and *Cool Cats, Calm Kids: Relaxation and Stress Management for Young People* (**Impact Publishing, 1996**).

Name: _____ Date: _____

WHAT IS SELF-ESTEEM?

Write True or False for each statement. If false, change the underlined word or phrase to make it true.

_____ 1. Talents and abilities that make us proud of ourselves are our <u>weaknesses</u>.

_____ 2. The qualities that make you different from everyone else are part of your <u>personality</u>.

_____ 3. If you have a good opinion of yourself, you will have a <u>positive</u> self-concept.

_____ 4. People with high self-esteem <u>often</u> get bored.

Write the word or phrase that best completes each sentence.

5. A person's basic physical needs include food, shelter, water, and

_____ .

6. You can build your self-esteem by choosing friends that have

_____ self-esteem.

7. An example of a health professional who can help rebuild a person's self-esteem is a _____ .

Answer each question with complete sentences.

8. What are two basic emotional needs that people have?

_____

9. How can knowing your strengths help build your self-esteem?

_____

_____

10. What are some signs that a person may need help rebuilding his or her self-esteem?

_____

_____

Name: _____   Date: _____

WHAT IS SELF-ESTEEM?

Complete the definition of each word.

1. Self-concept is _____

2. Personality is _____

3. Self-esteem is _____

4. Risk behaviors are _____

Answer each question in complete sentences.

5. What are three factors that influence the development of your personality?

   _____

6. What are some signs that a person has high self-esteem?

   _____

   _____

7. What is an example of a risk behavior that could be harmful to your social health?

   _____

8. What two choices can you make to strengthen your opinion of yourself?

   _____

   _____

9. How can high self-esteem affect physical health?

   _____

10. Who can you go to if you need help rebuilding your self-esteem?

    _____

    _____

Name: _____   Date: _____

EXPRESSING EMOTIONS

Write the word from the box that matches each picture.

| anger | fear | joy | sadness | sympathy | worry |

1. _____   2. _____   3. _____

4. _____   5. _____   6. _____

Answer each question with complete sentences.

7. How does expressing your emotions help your social health?

_____

8. What can you do if you think a conflict arose because of something you said?

_____

9. Who can help you resolve a conflict when nothing else seems to work?

_____

10. How can many misunderstandings be avoided?

_____

Name: _____   Date: _____

EXPRESSING EMOTIONS

Match the word or words in Column A with the description in Column B.
Write the correct letter in the blank.

Column A

_____ **1.** compromise

_____ **2.** conflict

_____ **3.** emotion

_____ **4.** resolution

Column B

A. a solution to a disagreement or struggle between people or ideas

B. to settle a disagreement or struggle by give and take

C. a strong feeling

D. a disagreement or struggle between people or ideas

Answer each question in complete sentences.

5. Which emotions are pleasant for you to feel? Which are uncomfortable?

_____

_____

6. How can keeping feelings bottled up affect a person's physical health?

_____

7. What are the benefits of calming down when dealing with conflict?

_____

8. What part does communication play in resolving conflicts?

_____

9. What should you do if a conflict is about to become violent? Why?

_____

10. What are some unhealthy ways of dealing with emotions?

_____

Name: _____ Date: _____

MANAGING STRESS

Here are five sentences about managing stress. Put a check mark in the blank beside each sentence that gives you good advice about dealing with stress or stressful situations. Then use complete sentences to explain why the advice is good or why it is not.

_____ **1.** Lie down, close your eyes, and relax by listening to some soothing music or by pretending you're in a quiet place.

_____

_____

_____ **2.** Don't worry about eating healthful foods or getting plenty of rest and sleep.

_____

_____

_____ **3.** Talk about your feelings with family members, friends, counselors, teachers, or other people you trust.

_____

_____

_____ **4.** Take a long walk or try some physical activity.

_____

_____

_____ **5.** Decide what to do about the stressful situation right away and take immediate action.

_____

_____

Name: _____   Date: _____

MANAGING STRESS

Write the word from the box that best completes each sentence.

| distress | stress | stressor | tension |

1. Your body and mind's response to changes around you is _____.

2. Stress that has negative and harmful effects is _____ .

3. A feeling like something is straining inside you is _____.

4. Anything that causes stress is a _____ .

Answer each question in complete sentences.

5. What are some things that could cause stress in your life?

_____

6. What is an example of healthful stress?

_____

7. What are some body signals that you are feeling stressed?

_____

8. Why do risk behaviors cause stress?

_____

_____

9. Joe is worrying about an ill parent. How can this stress harm his health?

_____

10. What steps can you take to make responsible decisions when under stress?

_____

_____

Name: _____   Date: _____

EMOTIONAL AND INTELLECTUAL HEALTH

Match the word or words in Column A with its definition in Column B.
Write the correct letter in the blank.

Column A

_____ 1. compromise

_____ 2. conflict

_____ 3. emotion

_____ 4. personality

_____ 5. resolution

_____ 6. risk behaviors

_____ 7. self-concept

_____ 8. self-esteem

_____ 9. stress

_____ 10. stressor

Column B

A. the qualities that make you a unique individual

B. actions that can be harmful to your health

C. what you think about yourself

D. a disagreement or struggle between people or ideas

E. anything that causes stress

F. to settle a conflict or disagreement by give and take

G. your body and mind's response to changes around you

H. a solution to a conflict

I. the level of respect you have for yourself

J. a strong feeling

Circle the letter of the best answer.

11. Suppose you're angry because your sister borrowed your favorite sweater without asking and then spilled ink all over it, ruining it. A healthful response would be to

    a. ruin something of your sister's

    b. keep your feelings about it bottled up

    c. calm down and talk with her about it

12. One way to relieve stress is to

    a. keep worrying about the situation

    b. work on a hobby

    c. get less sleep

Name: _____ Date: _____

EMOTIONAL AND INTELLECTUAL HEALTH

13. People with high self-esteem

    a. always think they're perfect

    b. usually keep themselves neat and clean

    c. never feel stress

14. An unhealthy way to respond to stress in your everyday life would be to

    a. engage in risk behaviors

    b. express your emotions honestly and clearly

    c. get help from a trusted adult

Write the word that will best complete each sentence.

15. When you respect the kind of person you are, you have a
_____ self-concept.

16. An example of a _____ that causes stress and physical harm
is smoking.

17. To resolve a conflict, you should communicate your feelings and try to find a
way to _____ .

Answer each question in complete sentences.

18. How can stress have a positive effect?

_____

_____

19. What might you do if you are feeling anxious before giving a speech?

_____

_____

20. How can you show other people that you care?

_____

_____

Extra Credit: On a separate piece of paper, outline a plan for how you would
handle a disagreement with a friend about what activity to do together after school.

McGraw-Hill School Division

Name: _____   Date: _____

Dear Parent or Guardian,

We are about to start **Chapter 4, Family and Social Health**, in which we will explore this Big Idea:

> Relationships with family members and friends have an important effect on your physical, emotional, intellectual, and social health.

Your child will be learning about

- healthy families and how families influence physical, emotional, intellectual, and social health
- maintaining healthy friendships and dealing with people of all ages
- maintaining healthy relationships with classmates and dealing with peer pressure
- how attitudes are formed and how they affect relationships with others

Help your child fill out the checklist below. Talk about how practicing ideas from the checklist can help strengthen your relationships with families, friends, and others.

Family and Social Health
Family Checklist

☐ Our family understands that there are different kinds of families.

☐ We know that in healthy families and other healthy relationships, members try to communicate, show understanding and support, and cooperate.

☐ When problems come up between friends or family members, we settle differences in healthful ways.

☐ Adults and children appreciate and realize the benefits of having relationships with people of all ages.

☐ We understand the difference between positive and negative peer pressure and practice saying "no" to negative peer pressure.

☐ We are aware that attitudes, such as tolerance, prejudice, and stereotyping, affect our relationships with others.

If you are interested in learning more about family and social health, a good resource is: **A Family of Values** (Andrews & McMeel, 1995).

Name: _____   Date: _____

HEALTHY FAMILY LIFE

Match the word or words in Column A with the description in Column B.
Write the correct letter in the blank.

Column A

_____ 1. extended family

_____ 2. single-parent family

_____ 3. adoptive family

_____ 4. nuclear family

_____ 5. blended family

Column B

A. a family adopts and raises children born to others

B. family includes other relatives who might act as parents

C. one or both parents have been married before; may include children from a previous marriage

D. one parent raises children

E. two parents raise children

Write True or False for each statement. If false, change the underlined word or phrase to make it true.

_____ 6. It's unusual for family members to argue sometimes.

_____ 7. In a healthy family, members try to communicate, show support, cooperate, and settle differences.

_____ 8. When you are dependable, it means that others cannot count on you.

_____ 9. A foster family cares temporarily for one or more children born to others.

Write complete sentences to answer the question.

10. How is a *privilege* different from a *right*?

_____

_____

Name: _____   Date: _____

HEALTHY FAMILY LIFE

Complete the definition of each word.

1. Dependability is _____

2. A privilege is _____

3. A relationship is _____

4. A responsibility is _____

5. A role is _____

Answer each question in complete sentences.

6. What are some roles your family members play?

   _____

   _____

7. How can praise and encouragement from family members affect your emotional health?

   _____

8. What can you learn about relationships with other people by being a member of a healthy family?

   _____

   _____

9. How does your family influence your physical health?

   _____

   _____

10. How can family members build trust and show respect for each other?

    _____

Name: _____   Date: _____

BUILDING HEALTHY RELATIONSHIPS

Underline the phrase that best completes each sentence.

1. A friend is someone who (ignores, understands) your feelings.

2. When trying to straighten things out with a friend, begin your sentences with (I, you).

3. A friend that joins a clique and leaves you out is acting in (a friendly, an unfriendly) way.

4. A friend fails to respect your feelings and beliefs over and over again. It is most likely time (to have an argument, to end the friendship).

5. Crying is an infant's way of (communicating with, annoying) people.

Answer each question in complete sentences.

6. What is one way you could meet new friends?

_____

7. What does it mean to appreciate a friend?

_____

8. Why are friends usually willing to compromise when there's a problem?

_____

9. What can you do when a friend acts unfriendly?

_____

_____

10. When you're around very young children, why should you pay careful attention to them?

_____

_____

McGraw-Hill School Division

Grade 5, Chapter 4, Lesson 2

Name: _____   Date: _____

BUILDING HEALTHY RELATIONSHIPS

Write the word from the box that best completes each sentence.

1. A small group whose members don't include others is a _____.

2. To recognize the value of a person or thing is to _____.

3. A person you share interests with and can count on is a _____.

Answer each question in complete sentences.

4. What is involved in being a good friend?

_____

_____

5. How would you stay close to a friend who has moved away?

_____

6. How can knowing how to listen help make you a good friend?

_____

_____

7. Why is it important to let friends know how you feel?

_____

8. In a healthy relationship, what do people do when they disagree?

_____

9. In what ways can older people be helpful friends to you?

_____

10. What are some things you can do to build your sense of responsibility when you're around young children?

_____

_____

Grade 5, Chapter 4, Lesson 2

Name: _____   Date: _____

PEER AND CLASSROOM RELATIONSHIPS

Write True or False for each statement. If false, change the underlined word or phrase to make it true.

_____ 1. When friends try to convince you to recycle, they are putting <u>positive</u> peer pressure on you.

_____ 2. Taking a stand against negative peer pressure is <u>never</u> difficult.

_____ 3. When friends pressure you to do something unhealthful, you <u>should</u> go along with them.

_____ 4. A student carries out his or her role <u>by learning</u>.

_____ 5. During a fire drill, you should <u>follow</u> your teacher's directions.

Answer each question in complete sentences.

6. What is one way to avoid situations that might cause you problems?

_____

7. Why is cooperation important in an effective classroom?

_____

Look at the picture. What are three things that show this is an effective classroom?

8. _____

_____

9. _____

_____

10. _____

_____

Name: _____   Date: _____

PEER AND CLASSROOM RELATIONSHIPS

Complete the definition of each word.

1. A peer is _____

2. Peer pressure is _____

3. Peer pressure is positive when it influences you to _____

4. Negative peer pressure tries to influence you to do things that are _____

5. Cooperation means that _____

Answer each question in complete sentences.

6. In what way is a healthy family and a healthy classroom alike?

_____

_____

7. Why is it sometimes difficult to take a stand against negative peer pressure?

_____

_____

_____

8. What are three things you are responsible for in the classroom?

_____

_____

_____

9. What should you do when someone tries to pressure you to do something unhealthful?

_____

_____

_____

10. Why is it important to be in charge of yourself?

_____

_____

_____

Name: _____ Date: _____

ATTITUDES AND RELATIONSHIPS

A family from another country moves in next door to you. They have a child who is your age and who will be in your class. The family members dress in their native clothing and have customs that are very different from yours.

Use a word from the box to identify each kind of attitude described below. Then use complete sentences to explain your answers.

| intolerance | prejudice | bossiness | stereotype | tolerance |

1. You decide to welcome the new family, make friends with the child, and try to learn more about their culture.

   _____

   _____

2. When your new neighbor comes to school the next day, the other kids in your class start making fun of how he looks and dresses.

   _____

   _____

3. A classmate says that *all* people from your neighbor's country dress weirdly.

   _____

   _____

4. A classmate is impolite to your new friend, though she doesn't know him. She says, "Those people don't deserve respect."

   _____

   _____

5. The leader of your after-school club never listens to your suggestions and gets angry when you ask him to repeat something.

   _____

   _____

Name: _____   Date: _____

ATTITUDES AND RELATIONSHIPS

Match the word or words in Column A with the description in Column B.
Write the correct letter in the blank.

Column A

_____ 1. tolerance

_____ 2. stereotype

_____ 3. prejudice

_____ 4. intolerant

_____ 5. attitude

Column B

A. an oversimplified image that assumes that all the members of a group have the same traits

B. an unfair opinion or judgment formed without knowing all the facts

C. a way of feeling and believing that affects your behavior

D. an ability to accept differences in people

E. not allowing for differences in others

Answer each question in complete sentences.

6. Why is it good to have a positive outlook and keep an open mind?

_____

7. As a member of a group, how can you help the group achieve its goals?

_____

_____

8. In what ways are your attitudes formed?

_____

_____

9. Why is it unfair to think of people in stereotypes?

_____

10. What are the characteristics of a good leader?

_____

_____

Name: _____   Date: _____

FAMILY AND SOCIAL HEALTH

Write the word from the box that best completes each sentence.

appreciate	attitude	clique	dependability	peer	responsibility
peer pressure	prejudice	privilege	relationship	role	tolerance

1. The quality of being reliable is _____.

2. Someone who is about the same age as you are is your _____.

3. To recognize the value of a person or thing is to _____.

4. The part someone plays is a _____.

5. An unfair opinion or judgment formed without knowing all the facts is
   _____.

6. A small group whose members stick together and don't include others is a
   _____.

7. A way of believing that affects your behavior is an _____.

8. A connection with another person or group is a _____ .

9. Social pressure from people your own age to act or think a certain way is
   _____.

10. A special favor or advantage is a _____.

11. An ability to accept differences in people is _____.

12. A job or a duty is a _____.

Circle the letter of the best answer.

13. If a friend promises to help you with your homework and then forgets to show up, you're most likely to feel

    a. disappointed   **b.** intolerant   **c.** peer pressure

14. The student sitting next to you in class doesn't feel well. You should

    a. walk away   **b.** tell your teacher immediately   **c.** be very quiet

Name: _____ Date: _____

FAMILY AND SOCIAL HEALTH

15. One way to offer support to friends and family members is to

    a. tell them what they're doing wrong

    b. ignore their thoughts and feelings

    c. attend events that are important to them

16. When one or both parents have been married before and each has children from a previous marriage, they form

    a. an extended family **b.** a nuclear family   **c.** a blended family

Answer each question in complete sentences.

17. In what ways can change strain a family?

_____

_____

18. How can interaction with your family affect your relationships with others?

_____

_____

19. How could you help out a friend who is an older person?

_____

20. In what ways can members of a healthy relationship show care and respect for each other?

_____

_____

Extra Credit: On a separate piece of paper, write a paragraph describing how your relationships with a friend or family member affects your physical, social, and emotional and intellectual health.

health

Name: _____   Date: _____

Dear Parent or Guardian,

We are about to start **Chapter 5, Nutrition**, in which we will explore this Big Idea:

> One can maintain health by eating a variety of nutritious foods, choosing healthful snacks, and maintaining a balanced diet.

Your child will be learning about

- what nutrients are and what happens to your body when it doesn't get the proper nutrients

- the Food Guide Pyramid and its use in planning meals for a balanced diet

- important guidelines to follow for a balanced diet and why too much fat in your diet is unhealthful

- the problems of fad diets and ways to maintain a healthful weight

Help your child fill out the checklist below. Talk about how practicing ideas from the checklist can help your family members maintain a proper diet.

Nutrition
Family Checklist

☐ Our family tries to maintain a schedule of three daily meals.

☐ We each try to drink six to eight glasses of water daily.

☐ We plan meals so that each family member has a balanced diet.

☐ Each family member participates in regular physical activity to maintain a healthful weight.

☐ We try to avoid snacks that have "empty" calories and few nutrients.

☐ We avoid fad diets and recognize the signs of eating disorders.

☐ We limit our consumption of saturated fats.

☐ We prevent food contamination by washing our hands when handling food and keeping cooking utensils and cutting boards clean.

If you are interested in learning more about nutrition, a good resource is: ***Diet and Nutrition Sourcebook,*** Dan Harris, ed. (Omnigraphics, 1996).

McGraw-Hill School Division

Name: _____   Date: _____

NUTRIENTS AND YOUR HEALTH

Write the word from the box that best completes each sentence.

calorie	carbohydrates	nutrients	proteins	vitamins

1. Substances in food that are needed to maintain health are

   _____ .

2. A unit that is used to measure the amount of energy in food is a

   _____ .

3. Nutrients that the body needs in small amounts to grow and function

   well are _____ .

4. Nutrients that provide materials for growth, maintenance, and repair

   of cells are _____ .

5. Nutrients that are the body's main source of energy are

   _____ .

Write True or False for each statement. If false, change the underlined word or phrase to make it true.

_____   6. There is no single "perfect" food that will give you all the nutrients your body needs.

_____   7. Sugar and starches are two main kinds of proteins.

_____   8. Minerals are nutrients that the body needs in small amounts to control body processes and build new cells.

_____   9. People can live only a few days without food.

_____   10. Anemia is a disease that may result from a diet with too little of the mineral iron.

Name: _____   Date: _____

NUTRIENTS AND YOUR HEALTH

Match the word in Column A with the description in Column B.
Write the correct letter in the blank.

Column A

_____ **1.** calorie

_____ **2.** carbohydrates

_____ **3.** nutrients

_____ **4.** protein

_____ **5.** vitamins

Column B

A. a unit that is used to measure the amount of energy in food

B. nutrients that provide materials for growth, maintenance, and repair of cells

C. nutrients that the body needs in small amounts to grow and function well

D. substances in food that are needed to maintain health

E. nutrients that are the body's main source of energy

Answer each question in complete sentences.

6. What are the functions of nutrients?

_____

7. What are the six categories of nutrients?

_____

8. Why should you drink six to eight glasses of water every day?

_____

9. The number of calories a person needs varies with what factors?

_____

10. Name a disease that is related to poor eating, and its cause.

_____

_____

Name: _____   Date: _____

FOOD GUIDE PYRAMID

Write the word or phrase from the box that best completes each sentence.

balanced diet	food groups
Food Guide Pyramid	recommended serving

1. Groups made up of foods that contain similar amounts of important nutrients are _____ .

2. The _____ is a diagram that provides information about food groups and healthful daily servings from each group.

3. A _____ is a suggested amount of food to eat to maintain a healthy diet.

4. A _____ is a diet, maintained over time, that includes a variety of foods that provide nutrition in moderate amounts.

Underline the word or phrase that best completes each sentence.

5. Fats, oils, and sweets should be used (often, sparingly).

6. The Bread, Cereal, Rice, and Pasta Group includes foods from (animals, grains).

7. Eating a balanced meal (is, is not) the same as having a balanced diet.

8. Fats, oils, and sweets have many calories and (few, many) nutrients.

9. A good source of fiber is the (Milk, Yogurt, Cheese Group; Vegetable Group).

10. The Bread, Cereal, Rice, and Pasta Group is a good source of (carbohydrates, fats).

McGraw-Hill School Division

Name: _____   Date: _____

FOOD GUIDE PYRAMID

1. Groups made up of foods that contain similar amounts of important nutrients are _____ .

2. A diagram that provides information about food groups and healthful daily servings from each group is the _____ .

3. Foods that should be used sparingly are _____ .

4. A diet maintained over time, that includes a variety of foods, providing nutrition in moderate amounts is a _____ .

5. The greatest number of servings in your diet each day should come from the _____ Group.

Answer each question in complete sentences.

6. Why is a balanced meal not the same as a balanced diet?

   _____

   _____

7. How does the Food Guide Pyramid help you plan a healthy diet?

   _____

8. What nutrient is supplied by the Bread, Cereal, Rice, and Pasta Group?

   _____

9. Why are Fats, Oils, and Sweets at the top of the Food Guide Pyramid?

   _____

   _____

10. What nutrients are supplied by the Milk, Yogurt, and Cheese Group?

   _____

McGraw-Hill School Division

Name: _____   Date: _____

MAKING FOOD CHOICES

Write <u>True</u> or <u>False</u> for each statement. If false, change the underlined word or phrase to make it true.

_____ 1. Availability of food at certain times of the year <u>may be a factor</u> that influences your food choices.

_____ 2. Keep your weight at a healthy level by balancing your food intake with <u>diets</u>.

_____ 3. Too much sugar can also lead to <u>tooth decay</u>.

_____ 4. Excess sugar is stored as body <u>muscle</u>.

_____ 5. No more than 30% (1/3) of your daily calories should come from <u>fats</u>.

_____ 6. <u>Vitamins</u> make the body store excess fluid which may result in weight gain and an increase in blood pressure.

_____ 7. "<u>Reduced Fat</u>" foods may have less fat than the original product, but they may still have many calories and a high fat content.

Write the word from the box that best completes each sentence.

media   saturated fat   unsaturated fat

8. A kind of fat, such as corn oil, most often made from plant-based foods is an _____ .

9. The _____ are forms of communication that reach a large audience.

10. A _____ is a kind of fat most often found in animal-based foods such as meat, cheese, and egg yolks.

McGraw-Hill School Division

Name: _____   Date: _____

MAKING FOOD CHOICES

1. Forms of communication that reach a large audience are the
   _____ .

2. A kind of fat, such as corn oil, most often made from plant-based
   foods is an _____ .

3. A kind of fat most often found in animal-based foods such as meat,
   cheese, and egg yolks is a _____ .

Answer each question in complete sentences.

4. How can the media influence your food choices?

   _____

5. How does the *Dietary Guidelines for Americans* issued by the
   U. S. Department of Agriculture help you?

   _____

   _____

6. How can you keep your weight at a healthy level?

   _____

7. Excess sugar can lead to what health problem?

   _____

8. Why should you avoid salty foods?

   _____

   _____

9. How can snacks contribute to a balanced diet?

   _____

10. Why should only 10% of your fat intake come from saturated fats?

    _____

Name: _____   Date: _____

FOOD LABELING

Write the word or phrase from the box that best completes each sentence.

| additive | ingredients | perishable | preservative | processed foods |

1. An additive to keep food from spoiling is a _____.

2. Substances that are mixed together to make foods are _____.

3. Foods to which substances have been added during canning, freezing, or drying them are _____.

4. Foods that are likely to spoil are _____.

5. An ingredient added to packaged food to improve its nutrient content is an _____.

Read the food label. Then underline the word that completes each sentence.

Nutrition Facts
Serving Size 1

Calories	80
	% DV*
Fat 0g	0%
Cholesterol 0mg	0%
Sodium 230mg	10%
Total Carb. 18g	6%
Fiber 1g	4%
Sugars 2g	
Protein 1g	

Vitamin A	10%	Vitamin C	15%
Calcium	0%	Iron	30%
Vitamin D	8%	Thiamin	15%

* Percent Daily Values (DV) are based on a 2,000 calorie diet.

Ingredients: Milled corn, sugar, salt, malt flavoring, high fructose corn syrup, ascorbic acid (vitamin C)

6. The number of servings is (1, 21).

7. The number of calories in one serving is (0, 80).

8. One serving of the product gives you (less, more) than the total Daily Value of sodium.

9. The nutrient with the highest Percent Daily Value is (iron, vitamin C).

10. There is more (corn syrup, milled corn) than any other ingredient.

Name: _____   Date: _____

FOOD LABELING

Match the word or phrase in Column A with the description in Column B.
Write the correct letter in the blank.

Column A

_____ **1.** additive

_____ **2.** ingredients

_____ **3.** perishable

_____ **4.** preservative

_____ **5.** processed foods

_____ **6.** expiration date

Column B

A. substances that are mixed together to make foods

B. an ingredient added to processed food to improve its taste

C. an additive that keeps food from spoiling quickly

D. the last day a food can be eaten safely

E. foods to which substances have been added during canning or freezing

F. likely to spoil within a short time

Answer each question in complete sentences.

7. Why are processed grain products enriched with vitamin B or iron?

_____

8. Why must food preservatives be listed on food labels?

_____

_____

9. Why should you never buy a product after its printed expiration date?

_____

10. How are the ingredients in a food package listed on the label?

_____

Name: _____   Date: _____

FOOD SAFETY HABITS

Write the word or phrase from the box that best completes each sentence.

botulism	contamination	food poisoning	Salmonella

1. A kind of bacteria that causes illness is _____.

2. Spoilage caused by unclean conditions is _____.

3. Food poisoning caused by toxins, or poisons, produced by certain bacteria is _____.

4. An illness caused by eating spoiled foods is

   _____.

Write True or False for each statement. If false, change the underlined word or phrase to make it true.

_____ 5. Salmonella are bacteria that grow on <u>uncooked</u> eggs and some meats.

_____ 6. Botulism is a rare illness that comes from <u>food</u> that has spoiled in a can or other container.

_____ 7. You can leave leftovers at room temperature for no more than <u>five</u> hours.

_____ 8. Buying food <u>before</u> its expiration date increases the risk of getting food that is spoiled.

_____ 9. You should keep refrigerated food at <u>a temperature of 40°F</u> or lower.

_____ 10. Sometimes, bacteria from one food item spoils other foods that are placed on the same <u>surface</u>.

Name: _____   Date: _____

FOOD SAFETY HABITS

Match the word or words in Column A with the description in Column B.
Write the correct letter in the blank.

Column A	**Column B**
_____ **1.** bacteria	**A.** spoilage caused by unclean conditions
_____ **2.** botulism	**B.** a kind of bacteria that causes illness
_____ **3.** contamination	**C.** tiny living organisms
_____ **4.** food poisoning	**D.** food poisoning caused by toxins, or poisons, produced by certain bacteria
_____ **5.** Salmonella	**E.** an illness caused by eating spoiled foods

Answer each question in complete sentences.

6. What are two types of organisms that can cause food poisoning?

_____

7. What should you do if you feel you've become sick from spoiled food?

_____

8. What are three signs of spoiled foods?

_____

_____

9. How can food contamination be avoided?

_____

_____

10. In what two ways can you store food so that it is safe to eat?

_____

_____

Name: _____   Date: _____

EATING HABITS AND YOUR HEALTH

Underline the word or phrase that best completes each sentence.

1. The key to maintaining a healthful body weight is to (burn up, store) the calories you take in from the food you eat.

2. Government guidelines state that boys and girls your age need between (220 and 250, 2200 and 2500) calories a day.

3. Sitting quietly uses (fewer, more) calories than jogging for the same amount of time.

4. Fad diets are usually unhealthful because they (limit people to eating certain foods, let people eat all types of food).

5. Stress and (low self-esteem, a positive attitude) may result in poor eating habits.

Write the word or phrase from the box that best completes each sentence.

anorexia nervosa	bulimia	caloric expenditure	caloric intake	fad diet

6. The calories a person burns up is _____.

7. An eating disorder in which a person eats large amounts of food in a short time and then vomits on purpose is _____.

8. A weight-loss diet that is popular and usually unhealthful is called a _____.

9. The number of calories a person consumes is called _____.

10. An eating disorder in which a person has an unrealistic fear of becoming overweight and eats very little is _____.

McGraw-Hill School Division

Name: _____ Date: _____

EATING HABITS AND YOUR HEALTH

Match the word or words in Column A with the description in Column B.
Write the correct letter in the blank.

Column A

_____ **1.** anorexia nervosa

_____ **2.** bulimia

_____ **3.** caloric expenditure

_____ **4.** caloric intake

_____ **5.** fad diet

Column B

A. the number of calories in the food a person eats

B. a weight-loss diet, popular for a short time; usually unhealthy

C. an eating disorder in which a person eats large amounts of food in a short time and then vomits on purpose

D. an eating disorder in which a person has an unrealistic fear of becoming overweight

E. the number of calories a person's body uses or burns up

Answer each question in complete sentences.

6. What is the key to maintaining a healthful body weight?

_____

7. What are some body functions that help burn calories?

_____

8. What is a problem with a diet that limits the type of food you eat?

_____

9. Why is bulimia dangerous to the body?

_____

10. What is one way of substituting low-fat foods for fatty foods?

_____

_____

McGraw-Hill School Division

Name: _____   Date: _____

NUTRITION

Write the word or phrase from the box that best completes each sentence.

additive	bulimia	balanced diet	botulism	saturated fat
calorie	food groups	unsaturated fat	nutrients	preservative

1. Substances in food that are needed for health are _____.

2. Unit used to measure the energy in food is the _____.

3. A diet that includes a variety of heathful foods is a _____.

4. Groups made up of foods that contain similar amounts of important nutrients are called _____.

5. A kind of fat made from plant-based foods is an _____.

6. Fat found mostly in animal-based foods is a _____.

7. An ingredient added to processed or packaged food to improve its taste is an _____.

8. When a _____ is added, food doesn't spoil quickly.

9. A food poisoning caused by certain bacteria is _____.

10. A person with _____ eats a lot of food and then vomits.

Circle the letter of the best answer.

11. A nutrient that carries other nutrients to your cells is

    a. calcium   **b.** fiber   **c.** water

12. Salt makes the body store excess fluid, resulting in increased

    a. saturated fat   **b.** cholesterol   **c.** weight gain

Name: _____   Date: _____

NUTRITION

13. The Daily Value listed on a food label shows

    a. the number of calories contained in each serving

    b. the most important ingredient contained in each serving

    c. the part of 100% of each nutrient contained in each serving

14. Balancing caloric intake with caloric expenditure is an effective way to

    a. exercise   **b.** increase body fat   **c.** maintain a healthy weight

15. Fats, oils, and sweets should be used sparingly because they supply

    a. "empty" calories   **b.** little water   **c.** too much iron

Answer each question in complete sentences.

16. On what factors does a healthful body weight depend?

_____

17. Why should your diet contain 6–11 servings from the Bread, Cereal, Rice, and Pasta food group every day?

_____

Write True or False for each statement. If false, change the underlined word or phrase to make it true.

_____ **18.** Both the Fruit Group and the Vegetable Group provide fiber in the daily diet.

_____ **19.** You should limit saturated fat because it has been linked to headaches.

_____ **20.** Food may be spoiled if it is sold after the expiration date marked on the package.

Extra Credit: On a separate piece of paper, write a paragraph that explains how poor eating habits may be related to a person's emotions.

Dear Parent or Guardian,

We are about to start **Chapter 6, Physical Activity and Fitness**, in which we will explore this Big Idea:

Regular physical activity will help your body perform at its best. It will also help you enjoy spending time with others and feel good about yourself.

Your child will be learning about

- the fitness skills that help you work, play, think, and feel
- the ways that these skills can be strengthened to improve fitness
- different types of physical activities
- ways to measure fitness and plan a fitness program
- how to stay safe during physical activity

Help your child fill out the checklist below. Talk about how practicing ideas from the checklist can help your family keep fit and feel better.

Physical Activity and Fitness
Family Checklist

☐ Our family engages in physical activities together, such as biking, walking, swimming, and skating.

☐ We try new physical activities to increase our fitness skills.

☐ Before engaging in physical fitness activities, we get ready with warm-up exercises.

☐ When we finish fitness activities we do cool-down activities that give our bodies a chance to recover.

☐ Our family chooses a variety of different types of exercise to promote physical fitness.

☐ We have specific fitness goals and check our progress using a family fitness program.

☐ Children and adults always use necessary safety equipment for physical activities.

☐ We know it is important to listen to our bodies for clues about when it is time to rest or slow down.

If you are interested in learning more about physical activity and fitness, a good resource is: **Sports Success from 6 to 16** by Michael Yessis (**Master Press, 1997**).

McGraw-Hill School Division

Name: _____   Date: _____

THE IMPORTANCE OF PHYSICAL FITNESS

Write the word from the box that best completes each sentence.

strength	body composition	posture
endurance		flexibility

1. You can increase your _____ by doing exercises that stretch your muscles and work your joints.

2. The amount of the body's fat tissue in relation to lean tissue is

   _____ .

3. Lifting a heavy box requires _____ .

4. Sitting erect in a chair or standing up straight are examples of good

   _____ .

5. The ability of your heart and lungs to keep you physically active without

   getting tired is called heart and lung _____ .

Write True or False for each statement. If false, change the underlined word or phrase to make it true.

_____ 6. Regular exercise can help you increase your resting heart rate.

_____ 7. Exercise can help your lungs get rid of more carbon dioxide.

_____ 8. To be healthy, your body needs no fat.

_____ 9. Working on physical fitness goals can help us make new friends.

_____ 10. Being physically fit helps produce stress.

Name: _____   Date: _____

THE IMPORTANCE OF PHYSICAL FITNESS

Match the word in Column A with the description in Column B.
Write the correct letter in the blank.

Column A

_____ **1.** body composition

_____ **2.** endurance

_____ **3.** flexibility

_____ **4.** physical fitness

_____ **5.** posture

_____ **6.** strength

Column B

A. the ability to lift, push, and pull

B. the ability to bend and move easily

C. the way a person holds his or her body

D. the ability to be active for a while without getting too tired to continue

E. the condition in which your body works at its best

F. the amount of fat tissue in relation to lean tissue in your body

Answer each question in complete sentences.

7. How can exercise benefit your heart?

_____

_____

8. Does exercise increase or decrease your lungs' efficiency? Explain.

_____

_____

9. How are exercise and body weight related?

_____

_____

10. In what ways can exercise improve emotional health?

_____

_____

Name: _____   Date: _____

FITNESS SKILLS

Underline the phrase that best completes each sentence.

1. Good (coordination, balance) helps your eyes work with your arm muscles when you throw a ball.

2. People who (remain physically active, avoid exercise) have better health.

3. Walking slowly through a tricky obstacle course can help you develop your (speed, agility)

4. You can improve your power by (jumping up and down, playing tug-of-war with a partner).

Write the word or words from the box that matches each pictured activity.

agility	balance	coordination	power	speed	reaction time

5.

_____

6.

_____

7.

_____

8.

_____

9.

_____

10.

_____

Name: _____   Date: _____

FITNESS SKILLS

Write the word or phrase that best completes each sentence.

1. The ability to make different parts of the body work well together to perform a task is _____ .

2. The ability to move and change position quickly and easily is _____ .

3. The combination of speed and strength produces _____ .

4. The ability to keep your body in a steady position is _____ .

5. Your ability to move quickly is your _____ .

6. The time it takes to notice and to respond to something is called _____ .

Answer each question in complete sentences.

7. What kinds of activities can agility help you do?

_____

_____

8. What fitness skill would you develop by practicing juggling?

_____

_____

9. Describe one way that you can develop your balance.

_____

_____

10. Explain whether or not reaction time is required when you play softball.

_____

_____

Name: _____   Date: _____

TYPES OF PHYSICAL ACTIVITY

Complete each sentence with a word from the box. One word will be used twice.

isometric	isotonic
aerobic	anaerobic

1. A push-up is an example of an _____ exercise because it uses muscle contraction and movement to build strength.

2. An _____ exercise uses up more oxygen than your heart and lungs can provide.

3. Jogging, in-line skating, and jumping rope are all examples of _____ exercises.

4. Pressing your hands against a door frame is an example of an _____ exercise because it builds strength using very little body movement.

5. An _____ exercise should be done briskly for about 20 to 30 minutes.

Write True or False for each statement. If false, change the underlined word or phrase to make it true.

_____ 6. Isometric exercises <u>cannot increase</u> muscle strength.

_____ 7. Aerobic exercise should be done at a medium or <u>moderately fast</u> pace.

_____ 8. An anaerobic exercise should be done for <u>at least 20 minutes</u>.

_____ 9. You should begin a workout with a <u>rapid aerobic</u> exercise.

_____ 10. Cool-down exercises can be a <u>fast</u> version of the workout exercise you were doing.

Name: _____   Date: _____

TYPES OF PHYSICAL ACTIVITY

Match the word in Column A with the description in Column B.
Write the correct letter in the blank.

Column A

_____ 1. aerobic exercise

_____ 2. anaerobic exercise

_____ 3. isometric exercise

_____ 4. isotonic exercise

Column B

A. an activity that is done briefly

B. a brisk and constant physical activity that increases the supply of oxygen

C. a physical activity that builds muscle strength and flexibility

D. an activity in which you strengthen muscles with little body movement

Answer each question in complete sentences.

5. If you make your hands into fists and squeeze tightly, what kind of exercise are you doing? What are some benefits of this exercise?

_____

6. How do isotonic exercises build physical fitness?

_____

7. What is an example of an aerobic activity, and what is it good for?

_____

8. How are anaerobic exercises different from aerobic exercises?

_____

_____

_____

9. How should you begin an exercise routine?

_____

10. How should you end an exercise routine?

_____

Name: _____   Date: _____

A PHYSICAL ACTIVITY PLAN

Here are some sentences about designing a physical activity plan. Put a check mark in the blank beside each sentence that gives you good advice about fitness. Then explain why each sentence is or is not good advice. Use complete sentences.

_____ **1.** It is impossible to measure how fit a person is.

_____

_____

_____

_____ **2.** A good fitness program should include a variety of activities instead of just one.

_____

_____

_____

_____ **3.** Warm-up exercises are only necessary if you are working out for more than 45 minutes.

_____

_____

_____

_____ **4.** A health journal can be a helpful fitness tool.

_____

_____

_____ **5.** It doesn't matter how often you exercise, so long as you exercise energetically when you do.

_____

_____

Name: _____   Date: _____

A PHYSICAL ACTIVITY PLAN

Write the word or phrase that best completes each sentence.

1. A good way for a person to measure his or her physical fitness is to take a _____ .

2. A good fitness test that can be used to measure your physical fitness is the _____ .

3. To reach long-term goals, it is a good idea to set _____ goals.

4. When I begin a fitness program, I should be aware of the FIT guidelines which stand for _____ .

Underline the phrase that best completes each sentence.

5. A good physical fitness program (does the right things in the right way, always increases).

6. It is important to maintain and improve (only the fitness skills that you lack, all basic physical fitness skills).

7. All fitness programs should include warm-up, workout, and (running, cool-down) exercises.

8. To maintain your physical fitness, you should exercise at least (three, nine) times a week.

9. You can measure the intensity of your workout by measuring your (height and weight, heart rate).

10. Your should gradually increase the length of each workout to about (five, thirty) minutes.

Name: _____ Date: _____

PHYSICAL ACTIVITY AND SAFETY

Complete each sentence with a word from the box.

blisters	safety equipment	flexible
injury		layers

1. When dressing for outdoor activities in cold weather, you should dress in

   _____ .

2. Harm or damage to a person or thing is an _____ .

3. Helmets and kneepads are types of _____ .

4. Some kneepads, such as those used by volleyball players, should be soft

   and _____ .

5. Cotton socks can be worn to cushion your feet and reduce

   _____ .

Write True or False for each statement. If false, change the underlined
word or phrase to make it true.

_____ 6. Water is the best thing to drink while
exercising.

_____ 7. Your exercise clothing should be loose
enough to let you move freely.

_____ 8. Rapid, high-energy exercises can help
prevent injury and soreness in your muscles.

_____ 9. Broken sporting equipment will protect you
as well as new equipment.

_____ 10. After exercise, your muscles should feel
worse than they did before you started.

Grade 5, Chapter 6, Lesson 5

Name: _____ Date: _____

PHYSICAL ACTIVITY AND SAFETY

Write the word or phrase that best completes each sentence.

1. Harm or damage to a person or thing is called _____ .

2. The best thing you can drink while exercising is _____ .

3. Being a _____ means respecting your opponents as well as your teammates.

4. Different materials designed to reduce the risk of injury are

   _____ .

Answer each question in complete sentences.

5. How tight should exercise clothing be?

   _____

6. What kinds of exercises can help prevent muscle injuries and soreness?

   _____

7. Why is it important to check sports equipment before you use it?

   _____

8. If you feel out of breath or unable to keep up a fast pace, what is your body telling you?

   _____

9. How can you be a good sport?

   _____

   _____

10. How do game rules help teams stay safe?

    _____

    _____

Name: _____ Date: _____

PHYSICAL ACTIVITY AND FITNESS

Write the word from the box that best completes each sentence.

```
body composition    safety equipment    injury    fitness test
isotonic    power    reaction    balance    aerobic    posture
```

1. The combination of speed and strength is _____ .

2. Your _____ time is the time it takes you to notice and to respond to something.

3. An _____ exercise is a physical activity that builds muscle strength and flexibility through muscle contraction and muscle movement.

4. Harm or damage to a person or thing is _____ .

5. The way a person holds her body while standing is _____ .

6. An _____ exercise is a brisk and constant physical activity that increases the supply of oxygen to your muscles.

7. The ability to keep your body in a steady position is _____ .

8. Materials designed to reduce the risk of injury are _____ .

9. The amount of fat tissue in relation to lean tissue in your body is your _____ .

10. The way to measure fitness is with a _____ .

Circle the letter of the best answer.

11. Being able to touch your toes requires
    a. strength   **b.** flexibility   **c.** coordination

12. To develop your coordination, you might
    a. hold your breath   **b.** play tug-of-war with a friend   **c.** learn to juggle

McGraw-Hill School Division

Name: _____   Date: _____

PHYSICAL ACTIVITY AND FITNESS

13. One example of an anaerobic exercise is

    a. bicycling   **b.** lifting weights   **c.** swimming

14. A good fitness program should include exercising about

    a. 3 times a week   **b.** 3 hours a day   **c.** 8 times a week

15. You can help prevent muscle injuries and soreness by doing

    a. aerobic exercises   **b.** warm-up exercises   **c.** isometric exercises

Answer each question in complete sentences.

16. How are strength and endurance different?

_____

_____

17. What is agility?

_____

18. How can you tell if an exercise is isometric or isotonic?

_____

_____

19. How should you choose exercises for a good physical fitness
program?

_____

_____

20. What should you think about before you use a piece of safety
equipment?

_____

Extra Credit: On a separate piece of paper, plan a fitness program that is meant
to improve your flexibility.

Name: _____ Date: _____

Dear Parent or Guardian,

We are about to start **Chapter 7, Disease Prevention and Control**, in which we will explore this Big Idea:

> Individuals can help prevent and control disease by knowing what causes disease, how diseases spread, how your body fights diseases, and what choices one can make to stay healthy.

Your child will be learning about

- communicable diseases and microbes that spread them
- preventing the spread of communicable disease
- how the body and its immune system protects against disease
- the effects of HIV on the immune system and ways of avoiding HIV infection and AIDS
- noncommunicable disease, their causes, and ways of lowering the risk of getting some of these diseases
- lifestyle choices and people who help you stay healthy

Help your child fill out the checklist below. Talk about how practicing ideas from the checklist can help your family members prevent and control diseases.

Disease Prevention and Control
Family Checklist

☐ Our family keeps antibacterial and antiseptic products in a first aid kit to prevent infections from burns and cuts.

☐ We wear proper protective clothing in areas where deer ticks may live.

☐ Family members have regular physical checkups.

☐ Family members are aware of and discuss risk factors concerning HIV and AIDS.

☐ Family members have received or are scheduled for the proper vaccinations and booster shots.

☐ Family members use sunscreens for protection against skin cancer.

☐ Family members are aware of and practice cleanliness as a means of preventing the spread of disease.

If you are interested in learning more about disease prevention and control, a good resource is: *Mosby's Handbook of Diseases* (Mosby, 1996).

Name: _____ Date: _____

LEARNING ABOUT DISEASES

Write the word from the box that best completes each sentence.

communicable disease	host	disease
noncommunicable disease	microbes	viruses

1. A breakdown in the way the body works is a _____ .

2. A disease that cannot be passed from person to person is a

   _____ .

3. A disease that is caused by microbes that invade the body is a

   _____ .

4. Microbes that can only reproduce inside living cells are

   _____ .

5. Antiseptics and antibacterial soaps kill _____ or keep

   them from growing.

6. The place that provides the environment in which microbes can live and

   reproduce is a _____ .

Write True or False for each statement. If false, change the underlined word or phrase to make it true.

_____ 7. A noncommunicable disease may be caused by underlined{heredity}.

_____ 8. As a virus uses substances in a cell to reproduce, it often underline{helps} the cell it has infected.

_____ 9. Athlete's foot is a disease caused by a underline{virus}.

_____ 10. Microbes are carried into the underline{air} when an infected person sneezes or coughs.

Name: _____   Date: _____

LEARNING ABOUT DISEASES

Match the word or words in Column A with the description in Column B.
Write the correct letter in the blank.

Column A

_____ 1. communicable disease

_____ 2. disease

_____ 3. microbe

_____ 4. noncommunicable disease

_____ 5. viruses

Column B

A. a breakdown in the way the body works

B. the tiniest pieces of living matter that reproduce inside a living cell

C. a disease that is not spread from one living thing to another

D. a tiny form of life, visible only with a microscope

E. a disease caused by microbes that can be passed to a person from another person, an animal, or an object

Answer each question in complete sentences.

6. What causes noncommunicable diseases?

_____

7. What causes communicable diseases?

_____

8. What are some types of disease-causing microbes?

_____

9. How are disease-causing microbes carried?

_____

_____

10. Why should you keep antibacterial soap in your family's first aid kit?

_____

_____

McGraw-Hill School Division

Grade 5, Chapter 7, Lesson 1

87

Name: _____   Date: _____

COMMUNICABLE DISEASES

Write the word or phrase from the box that best completes each sentence.

antibiotics	incubation	
influenza	symptom	vaccine

1. A communicable disease starts with an _____ period, before a person is even aware of being ill.

2. An indication of a disease is a _____.

3. Viruses cause the respiratory disease called _____.

4. A substance made from dead or weakened microbes that is injected or swallowed to protect the body against a specific disease is a

   _____.

5. Medicines that can kill bacteria are _____.

Underline the phrase that best completes each sentence.

6. During the (convalescent, peak) period of a communicable disease, you are recovering from the disease.

7. Influenza symptoms are similar to (cold, tetanus) symptoms—but worse.

8. Needle inoculation means you receive MMR and DPT vaccines by (injection, swallowing it).

9. To make vaccines, viruses are often grown on animal (tissue, waste products) in laboratories.

10. Washing hands, keeping flies away from food, and separating sick patients are changes in (behavior, heredity) that have helped to reduce diseases.

Name: _____   Date: _____

COMMUNICABLE DISEASES

Match the word in Column A with the description in Column B.
Write the correct letter in the blank.

Column A

_____ **1.** antibiotics

_____ **2.** incubation

_____ **3.** influenza

_____ **4.** symptom

_____ **5.** vaccine

Column B

A. a respiratory disease caused by a flu virus

B. medicines that kill bacteria

C. a substance made from dead or weakened microbes that protects the body against a specific disease

D. an indication of a disease

E. the period of a communicable disease when microbes grow inside the body's cells

Answer each question in complete sentences.

6. How can you "catch" a cold?

_____

7. How can diseases that are caused by bacteria living in water be prevented?

_____

8. How might you be able to avoid Lyme diseases?

_____

9. How can disease-causing bacteria be prevented from growing in food products?

_____

10. How are vaccines produced?

_____

_____

Name: _____   Date: _____

THE IMMUNE SYSTEM

Write the word or phrase from the box that best completes each sentence.

antibody	fever	immune system
immunity	white blood cells	

1. A raised body temperature — 99.6°F (37.7°C) or higher — is a
   _____.

2. All of the parts and functions of your body that fight disease-causing
   microbes make up your body's _____ .

3. A chemical made by the body that helps destroy or weaken bacteria,
   viruses, and other microbes is an _____.

4. Large blood cells that help the body fight disease are
   _____.

5. The protection against or ability to fight disease is _____.

Write True or False for each statement. If false, change the underlined
word or phrase to make it true.

_____   6. Your skin is the first line of defense to keep
                               disease-causing microbes from entering
                               your body.

_____   7. Your windpipe and all other air passages are
                               filled with cilia that constantly sweep
                               downward to prevent bacteria from entering
                               the lungs.

_____   8. Red blood cells stop the spread of disease
                               by surrounding microbes that enter the body.

_____   9. If you have immunity to a disease, you
                               probably will get the disease again.

_____   10. A vaccine contains a weakened or dead form
                               of a microbe that is not strong enough to
                               cause the disease, but is strong enough to
                               stimulate the production of an antibody.

Name: _____   Date: _____

THE IMMUNE SYSTEM

Match the word or words in Column A with the description in Column B.
Write the correct letter in the blank.

Column A

_____ 1. antibody

_____ 2. fever

_____ 3. immune system

_____ 4. immunity

_____ 5. white blood cells

Column B

A. protection against or ability to fight a disease

B. all of the parts and functions of your body that fight disease-causing microbes

C. a raised body temperature

D. blood cells that help the body fight disease

E. chemicals made by the body that help destroy harmful microbes

Answer each question in complete sentences.

6. What organ prevents disease-causing microbes from entering the body?

   _____

7. How do white blood cells stop the spread of disease?

   _____

8. How can a fever help fight a disease?

   _____

   _____

9. How do antibodies help produce immunity?

   _____

   _____

   _____

10. Why is it difficult to make a vaccine against the common cold, which is caused by many different types of viruses?

   _____

McGraw-Hill School Division

Name: _____ Date: _____

HIV AND AIDS

Write True or False for each statement. If false, change the underlined word or phrase to make it true.

_____ 1. HIV is a virus that causes a deficiency in the <u>nervous</u> system.

_____ 2. People with AIDS often become ill with tuberculosis or a very unusual type of <u>skin cancer</u>.

_____ 3. HIV <u>is</u> spread through casual contact.

_____ 4. Sexual contact is a <u>risk factor</u> for transmitting HIV.

_____ 5. HIV <u>can</u> be passed from the infected blood of an injured person.

Write the word or phrase from the box that best completes each sentence.

abstinence	AIDS	HIV
risk factor		syndrome

6. A virus that causes a deficiency in the immune system and leads to AIDS is _____.

7. The act of avoiding a behavior completely is _____ .

8. A group of symptoms that occur together in a particular disease is a _____.

9. A very serious disease in which the immune system is extremely weak is _____.

10. A trait or behavior that increases a person's chances of getting a disease is a _____.

McGraw-Hill School Division

Name: _____   Date: _____

HIV AND AIDS

Match the word or words in Column A with the description in Column B.
Write the correct letter in the blank.

Column A

_____ 1. abstinence

_____ 2. AIDS

_____ 3. HIV

_____ 4. risk factor

_____ 5. syndrome

Column B

A. a trait or behavior that increases a person's chance of getting a disease

B. a virus that can lead to AIDS

C. the act of avoiding a certain behavior

D. a group of symptoms that occur together in a particular disease

E. a disease, caused by infection with HIV

Answer each question in complete sentences.

6. How does HIV affect the immune system?

_____

_____

7. What three conditions exist when a person has AIDS?

_____

_____

8. In what three ways is HIV transmitted?

_____

_____

_____

9. Why is giving blood at a blood center not a risk factor in transmitting HIV?

_____

10. In what way can HIV infection be avoided?

_____

Name: _____   Date: _____

NONCOMMUNICABLE DISEASES

Underline the word or phrase that best completes each sentence.

1. One treatment of cancer is radiation, which uses (a form of high energy X-rays, very strong drugs) to kill cancer cells.

2. The leading cause of death in the United States is (cancer, heart disease).

3. If blood flow to the brain is blocked, a person may suffer a (heart attack, stroke).

4. Sickle cell anemia is a disease caused by (behavior, heredity).

5. Sunscreens help to protect you from (lung, skin) cancer.

Answer each question in complete sentences.

6. What causes noncommunicable diseases?

_____

_____

7. What is a chronic disease?

_____

_____

8. What is a degenerative disease?

_____

9. What is cancer?

_____

_____

10. What is a disease that is related to smoking?

_____

Name: _____   Date: _____

NONCOMMUNICABLE DISEASES

Match the word or words in Column A with the description in Column B.
Write the correct letter in the blank.

Column A

_____ 1. allergies

_____ 2. cancer

_____ 3. chemotherapy

_____ 4. chronic

_____ 5. degenerative

Column B

A. a treatment which uses very strong drugs to kill cancer cells

B. responses by the immune system to certain substances

C. lasting for a long time or coming back again and again

D. tending to get worse and worse

E. a disease that is caused when cells divide and multiply in ways that are not normal

Answer each question in complete sentences.

6. What is an example of a chronic disease?

_____

7. What is an example of a degenerative disease?

_____

8. What is a treatment for cancer?

_____

_____

9. What is the leading cause of death in the United States?

_____

10. What is one way to lower your risk of noncommunicable diseases?

_____

_____

Name: _____ Date: _____

STAYING HEALTHY

Label each pictured lifestyle choice that helps you stay healthy.

1.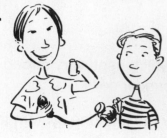

_____

2.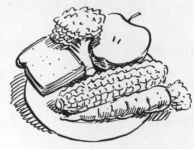

_____

3.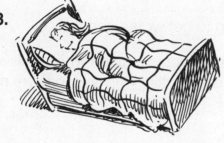

_____

4.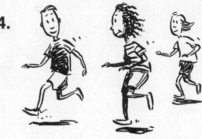

_____

Write True or False for each statement. If false, change the underlined word or phrase to make it true.

_____ 5. A lifestyle choice is a decision that affects the kind of life you live.

_____ 6. Smoking is a healthy lifestyle choice.

_____ 7. Resistance is your body's ability to fight off a disease.

_____ 8. Staying relaxed seems to have a good effect on the immune system.

_____ 9. Dieticians are responsible for preparing medicines that have been prescribed.

_____ 10. A food inspector makes sure that food is safe to eat.

Name: _____   Date: _____

STAYING HEALTHY

Write the word or phrase that best completes each sentence.

1. People who are responsible for preparing and providing medicines that have been prescribed by doctors for their patients are _____ .

2. Your body's ability to fight off a disease is _____ .

3. Decisions that affect the kind of life you lead are _____ .

4. If your _____ is functioning properly, your body will be resistant to disease.

5. A person who checks food to make sure it is fresh and free of harmful microbes and chemicals is a _____ .

Answer each question in complete sentences.

6. Why is it important to keep your immune system healthy?

_____

7. In what way can you keep your immune system healthy?

_____

_____

8. Why is it a good lifestyle choice to tell your parents or a trusted adult if you have symptoms of an illness?

_____

9. What is one task of a medical laboratory technologist?

_____

_____

_____

10. How does a dietician help keep people healthy?

_____

_____

Name: _____   Date: _____

DISEASE PREVENTION AND CONTROL

Write the word or phrase from the box that best completes each sentence.

AIDS	antibody	cancer	HIV	vaccine	symptom
communicable disease		immunity	microbe	resistance	

1. A virus that affects the immune system and can lead to AIDS is _____.

2. A disease caused by microbes that can be passed to a person, an animal, or an object is a _____ .

3. An indication of a disease is a _____ .

4. A disease in which cells multiply in abnormal ways is _____ .

5. A tiny form of life, visible only with a microscope, is a _____ .

6. A substance that is injected to protect the body against a specific disease is a _____ .

7. The protection against or ability to fight a disease is _____ .

8. Your body's ability to fight off a disease is called _____ .

9. A chemical made by the body that helps destroy or weaken bacteria, viruses, and other microbes is an _____ .

10. A serious disease caused by infection with HIV is _____ .

Circle the letter of the best answer.

11. Influenza is a disease caused by
    a. bacteria   **b.** fungi   **c.** viruses

12. Diabetes is a disease caused by
    a. behavior   **b.** heredity   **c.** mold

Name: _____   Date: _____

DISEASE PREVENTION AND CONTROL

13. The first known vaccine was used to fight

    a. cholera   **b.** small pox   **c.** diabetes

14. An intelligent way to prevent HIV infection is abstinence from sexual contact and from

    a. drug use   **b.** casual contact   **c.** smoking

15. The leading cause of death in the United States is

    a. cancer   **b.** emphysema   **c.** heart disease

Answer each question in complete sentences.

16. How does HIV affect the immune system?

_____

_____

17. How do you develop immunity against a particular microbe?

_____

_____

Write <u>True</u> or <u>False</u> for each statement. If false, change the underlined word or phrase to make it true.

_____ **18.** <u>Measles</u> is a communicable disease.

_____ **19.** Your <u>heart</u> is the main barrier between you and microbes.

_____ **20.** Some vaccines require a <u>booster</u> because the immunity lasts for only a few years.

Extra Credit: On a separate piece of paper, write a paragraph that explains three ways in which HIV is transmitted.

Name: _____   Date: _____

Dear Parent or Guardian,

We are about to start **Chapter 8, Alcohol, Tobacco, and Drugs,** in which we will explore this Big Idea:

> Drugs can be used wisely to prevent, cure, or treat illnesses. However, when misused or abused, drugs can have many harmful effects.

> Your child will be learning about

• legal and illegal drugs

• how addictive drugs can lead to drug dependence

• the health dangers of alcohol, tobacco, and illegal drugs

• the benefits of choosing a lifestyle that is free of tobacco, alcohol, and illegal drugs

Help your child fill out the checklist below. Talk about how practicing ideas from the checklist can help your family approach drugs carefully and wisely.

Alcohol, Tobacco, and Drugs
Family Checklist

☐ Our family takes special care whenever using medicine.

☐ We always read medicine labels and follow the recommended dosages.

☐ If a problem or question arises while taking a medicine, we contact our physician right away.

☐ We discuss the dangers of using tobacco and alcohol.

☐ We talk about the benefits of staying drug free.

☐ If we think that someone has a problem with alcohol or drugs, we recommend that they seek help or support.

☐ Our family has noticed the relationship between violence and drug use, and we talk about how staying drug free can help make everyone safer and healthier.

☐ We support our community through obeying laws regarding drug use.

If you are interested in learning more about alcohol and drug use, a good resource is: *Kids, Alcohol, and Drugs* **(Ballantine Books, 1991).**

Name: _____   Date: _____

LEGAL DRUGS AND ILLEGAL DRUGS

Write <u>True</u> or <u>False</u> for each statement. If false, change the underlined word or phrase to make it true.

_____   1. Drugs <u>cannot</u> do serious harm to your health.

_____   2. <u>Over-the counter</u> drugs can be purchased without a doctor's prescription.

_____   3. <u>Only illegal</u> drugs can have side effects.

_____   4. Illegal drugs may affect your <u>heart rate, blood pressure, and nervous system.</u>

_____   5. If a medicine is not working, you should <u>take twice the recommended dosage.</u>

Underline the phrase that best completes each sentence.

6. You must always get a doctor's written order when you need a (prescription, non-prescription) drug.

7. Alcohol and tobacco are examples of legal drugs that are not (dangerous, medicines).

8. The careless or improper use of a medicine or legal drug in a way that can harm you is (drug abuse, drug misuse).

9. The purposeful use of drugs in ways that can seriously harm your physical, emotional, intellectual, and social health is (drug abuse, drug misuse).

10. People who are caught with (over-the-counter, illegal) drugs can be sent to prison.

Name: _____   Date: _____

LEGAL DRUGS AND ILLEGAL DRUGS

Match the word or words in Column A with the description in Column B.
Write the correct letter in the blank.

Column A

_____ 1. drug

_____ 2. side effect

_____ 3. over-the-counter drug

_____ 4. prescription

_____ 5. drug abuse

Column B

A. a written order for medicine from a doctor

B. the purposeful use of drugs, particularly illegal drugs, in ways that can seriously harm your health

C. unwanted result of taking a medicine

D. a substance that causes changes in the body and mind

E. a drug that can be purchased without a doctor's prescription

Write the word from the box that best completes each sentence.

illegal	always	allergy
medicine		never

6. A drug that is used to prevent, treat, or cure illness is a

   _____ .

7. If someone has an _____ , that person is sensitive to certain substances.

8. You should _____ take a medicine that was prescribed for someone else.

8. Marijuana, cocaine, heroin, and amphetamines are examples of

   _____ drugs.

10. It is _____ important to follow directions when taking medicine.

Name: _____   Date: _____

DRUG DEPENDENCE

Here are some sentences about drug dependence. Put a check mark in the blank beside each sentence that gives you good advice about drugs. Then explain why each sentence is or is not good advice. Use complete sentences.

_____ **1.** Drug dependence can seriously harm a person's physical, intellectual and emotional, and social health.

_____

_____

_____

_____ **2.** Peer pressure is usually harmless because your peers always want the same things you do.

_____

_____

_____ **3.** You will never have to face the difficulties of withdrawal if you don't start taking drugs in the first place.

_____

_____

_____

_____ **4.** Becoming an active member of your community is a good strategy for staying drug free.

_____

_____

_____ **5.** When people have problems with drugs, they should try to solve their own problems without getting help from others.

_____

_____

_____

McGraw-Hill School Division

Name: _____   Date: _____

DRUG DEPENDENCE

Write the word or phrase that best completes each sentence.

1. When a person is _____ dependent on a drug, he or she believes that getting along in the world is impossible without the drug.

2. When a person is _____ dependent on a drug, he or she feels sick if the drug isn't present in the body.

3. The physical and emotional effects that occur when a drug user tries to stop using drugs is called _____.

4. The uncontrollable need to use a substance that is known to be unhealthful is called an _____.

5. When people use a drug over an extended period, they build up a _____.

Answer each question in complete sentences.

6. How can drug dependence affect a person's emotional and intellectual health?

   _____

   _____

7. What is an overdose?

   _____

   _____

8. How can your choice of friends help you stay drug free?

   _____

9. How can a person resist peer pressure?

   _____

   _____

10. How could you get help for someone who has a problem with drugs?

   _____

   _____

McGraw-Hill School Division

Grade 5, Chapter 8, Lesson 2   **105**

Name: _____ Date: _____

TOBACCO AND HEALTH

Underline the phrase that best completes each sentence.

1. The addictive drug in tobacco is (nicotine, carbon monoxide).

2. A substance that causes cancer is called a (poisonous gas, carcinogen).

3. Smoking increases the amount of (oxygen, carbon monoxide) in blood.

4. The (atherosclerosis, tar) in cigarette smoke contains many substances that are known to cause cancer.

5. Emphysema is a lung disease that prevents the body from getting enough (oxygen, nicotine).

Answer each question in complete sentences.

6. How does nicotine affect the heart?

_____

_____

7. What happens when carbon monoxide enters the blood?

_____

8. How are smoking and cancer related?

_____

Look at the picture. What are the benefits of staying tobacco free?

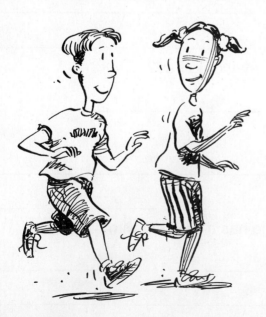

9. _____

_____

_____

_____

10. _____

_____

_____

Name: _____   Date: _____

TOBACCO AND HEALTH

Write the word or phrase that best completes each sentence.

1. When tobacco burns, a poisonous gas called _____ is produced.

2. A dark sticky mixture of chemicals called _____ is also found when tobacco burns.

3. A substance that causes cancer is called a _____.

4. Tobacco contains _____, a drug that speeds up the heart and causes addiction.

5. Smoking is the main cause of _____, a lung disease that prevents the body from getting enough oxygen.

Write True or False for each statement. If false, change the underlined word or phrase to make it true.

_____   6. When carbon monoxide enters the blood, it increases the amount of oxygen the blood can carry.

_____   7. Nonsmokers are less likely to have heart attacks than smokers.

_____   8. Smoking and using smokeless tobacco are addictive.

_____   9. One physical benefit of staying tobacco free is that you will have fewer colds and respiratory problems.

_____   10. One social benefit of staying tobacco free is that you will have less money to spend on other activities.

Name: _____   Date: _____

TOBACCO AND SOCIAL ISSUES

Here are some sentences about tobacco and social issues. Put a check mark in the blank beside each sentence that is true about smoking. Then explain why each sentence is or is not true. Use complete sentences.

_____ **1.** You can't be hurt by being with other people who smoke.

_____

_____

_____

_____ **2.** The Surgeon General has not found any evidence that smoking and cancer are related.

_____

_____

_____

_____ **3.** No-smoking laws help to keep public spaces safe and free of hazardous smoke.

_____

_____ **4.** Cigarette advertisements are required to show you the problems that can result from smoking.

_____

_____

_____

_____ **5.** Passive smoke is a threat to the lives of both children and adults.

_____

_____

_____

Name: _____ Date: _____

TOBACCO AND SOCIAL ISSUES

Complete the definition of each word.

1. Passive smoke is _____
   _____

2. The Surgeon General is _____
   _____

Underline the phrase that best completes each sentence.

3. More than two thirds of the adults in the United States (smoke, do not smoke).

4. Young children whose parents smoke often develop (resistance to nicotine, breathing problems).

5. Passive smoke (is the same as, is more serious than) environmental tobacco smoke.

6. Smoking is a serious health risk for (smokers only, both smokers and non-smokers).

Answer each question in complete sentences.

7. What is one short-term effect of passive smoke?
   _____

8. What is one long-term effect of passive smoke?
   _____
   _____

9. How do no-smoking laws help protect non-smokers?
   _____

10. What law helps to restrict the appeal of tobacco advertisements?
    _____
    _____

Name: _____   Date: _____

ALCOHOL AND THE FAMILY

Write the word from the box that best completes each sentence.

sober	withdrawal	alcoholism	intoxication	cirrhosis

1. An addiction to alcohol is called _____.

2. Drinking alcohol can lead to _____, a condition in which a person's coordination and judgment can be damaged.

3. Alcoholics Anonymous is a group that helps people stay _____.

4. Once physical dependence has set in, a person who tries to stop drinking may suffer painful _____.

5. Liver damage may lead to_____, a life-threatening disease that destroys healthy cells in the liver.

Underline the phrase that best completes each sentence.

6. Alcohol (increases, decreases) a person's ability to think and solve problems.

7. The (liver, heart) does most of the work of breaking down alcohol.

8. Leading an alcohol-free lifestyle can increase your (level of intoxication, control of your body and mind).

Describe a response to both of the following situations.

9. A friend's older brother offers you a beer.

_____

10. Your neighbor is worried that her cousin has a drinking problem.

_____

_____

McGraw-Hill School Division

Name: _____   Date: _____

ALCOHOL AND THE FAMILY

Write the word or phrase that best completes each sentence.

1. When a person is _____, his or her reaction time and judgment are seriously affected by alcohol.

2. When a person is _____, he or she is not under the influence of alcohol or any other mood-altering drug.

3. An addiction to alcohol is called _____.

4. One well-known recovery program for people who are addicted to alcohol is _____.

Answer each question in complete sentences.

5. What are two short-term effects of drinking alcohol?

_____

6. What is cirrhosis?

_____

7. Can drinking alcohol have long-term effects on the brain? Explain.

_____

8. How can drinking alcohol affect a person's self-esteem?

_____

_____

9. How can a person's social health be affected by drinking alcohol?

_____

_____

10. What are two benefits of an alcohol-free lifestyle?

_____

_____

McGraw-Hill School Division

Name: _____ Date: _____

MARIJUANA AND OTHER DRUGS

Complete the definition of each word.

1. A stimulant is _____

_____

2. An inhalant is _____

_____

3. A depressant is _____

_____

4. Marijuana is _____

_____

5. An amphetamine is _____

_____

Write True or False for each statement. If false, change the underlined word or phrase to make it true.

_____ 6. Marijuana interferes with the ability to think clearly.

_____ 7. Cocaine, coffee, and diet pills are all types of depressants.

_____ 8. All stimulants are highly addictive.

_____ 9. Inhaling fumes from glue or paint thinner can strengthen muscles and appetite.

_____ 10. Over-the-counter sleeping pills are never habit-forming.

Grade 5, Chapter 8, Lesson 6

Name: _____   Date: _____

MARIJUANA AND OTHER DRUGS

Match the word or words in Column A with the best description in Column B.
Write the correct letter in the blank.

Column A

_____ **1.** inhalant

_____ **2.** amphetamine

_____ **3.** depressant

_____ **4.** stimulant

_____ **5.** marijuana

Column B

A. a substance that gives off dangerous gases that can be inhaled

B. a drug that speeds up actions of the body and mind

C. a drug made from the hemp or cannabis plant

D. a stimulant that is very dangerous and leads to addiction

E. a drug that slows down actions of the body and mind

Answer each question in complete sentences.

6. How can using marijuana affect a person's thinking?

_____

7. Why is it hard to stop using stimulants?

_____

8. How are depressants different from stimulants?

_____

9. Are all over-the-counter medicines harmless? Explain.

_____

_____

10. What are some long-term effects of using inhalants?

_____

_____

Name: _____ Date: _____

NARCOTICS AND HALLUCINOGENS

Write the word from the box that best completes each sentence..

intravenous	HIV	hallucinogen
healthy		narcotics

1. A drug is _____ if the user injects it into the body with a needle.

2. A drug is a _____ if it makes the user see or hear things that are not really there.

3. Sharing needles can lead to the spread of the _____ virus.

4. Some drugs that are prescribed by doctors for sleep and to relieve pain are called _____.

5. Staying drug free can help you enjoy _____ relationships with family and friends.

Underline the phrase that best completes each sentence.

6. Heroin is an (illegal narcotic, legal amphetamine) that is very addictive and dangerous.

7. Withdrawal from heroin is very (quick and painless, difficult and painful).

8. People who use hallucinogens increase the risk of (lung or heart disease, accidents or overdose).

9. If your lifestyle choice is to remain drug free, you will be able to (act more violently, think clearly).

10. With a drug-free lifestyle, you most likely will take good care of yourself and have (high, low) self-esteem.

Name: _____   Date: _____

NARCOTICS AND HALLUCINOGENS

Write the word or phrase that best completes each sentence.

1. A drug that causes a person to see or hear things that are not really there is a _____.

2. A drug that enters the body by way of a vein is an _____.

3. A drug that produces sleep and dulls pain is a _____.

4. Drugs users develop an _____ to or dependence on narcotics very quickly.

Answer each question in complete sentences.

5. How can using drugs lead to HIV infection?

    _____

    _____

6. What is heroin?

    _____

7. How can heroin damage a person's health?

    _____

8. How can staying drug free help your schoolwork?

    _____

9. Can staying drug free help you avoid violence? Explain.

    _____

    _____

10. How can a drug-free lifestyle affect your self-esteem?

    _____

    _____

Name: _____ Date: _____

ALCOHOL, TOBACCO, AND DRUGS

Write the word from the box that best completes each sentence.

stimulant	addiction	carcinogen	intravenous	passive
withdrawal	intoxication	tar	prescription	depressant

1. A substance that causes cancer is a _____.

2. A drug that speeds up the mind and body is a _____.

3. A person has an _____ when he or she has an uncontrollable need to use a substance that is known to be unhealthful.

4. A drug that is _____ enters the body by way of a vein.

5. A drug that slows down the mind and body is a _____.

6. Tobacco smoke that is inhaled by nonsmokers is _____ smoke.

7. The mixture of chemicals in burning tobacco is called _____.

8. A written order for medicine from a doctor is a _____.

9. The effects of trying to quit drugs is called _____.

10. A person's coordination may be affected by _____.

Circle the letter of the best answer.

11. The purposeful use of drugs in harmful ways is

   a. drug abuse   b. hallucination   c. inhalation

12. To use an over-the-counter drug, you do not need to

   a. get a prescription   b. follow directions   c. read the label

13. Recovery programs for alcoholism help people stay

   a. tobacco free   b. sober   c. intoxicated

Name: _____   Date: _____

ALCOHOL, TOBACCO, AND DRUGS

14. Lung and heart disease are health problems associated with

    a. tobacco   **b.** sugar   **c.** prescriptions

15. A drug-free lifestyle encourages

    a. low self-esteem   **b.** weight loss   **c.** high self-esteem

Answer each question in complete sentences.

16. Are over-the-counter medicines always safe to use? Explain.

_____

17. How do laws help to protect people from the harmful effects of tobacco?

_____

_____

18. What can a person do to get help for an addiction to alcohol?

_____

19. How can using marijuana affect your intellectual health?

_____

_____

20. How can drug use lead to the spread of the HIV virus?

_____

_____

Extra Credit: Someone you know says that there are no positive reasons for choosing to be drug free. On a separate sheet of paper, write a response.

Name: _____   Date: _____

Dear Parent or Guardian,

We are about to start **Chapter 9, Safety, Injury, and Violence Prevention**, in which we will explore this Big Idea:

> Most injuries can be prevented by following safety rules, avoiding hazards, and asking for help when needed.

Your child will be learning about

- preventing injuries and maintaining a safe environment
- resolving conflicts and avoiding violence
- staying safe indoors and outdoors
- preventing fires and following fire safety precautions
- handling minor injuries and emergency situations

Help your child fill out the checklist below. Talk about how practicing ideas from the checklist can help your family stay safe from injury.

Safety, Injury, and Violence Prevention
Family Checklist

☐ Our family looks for hazards in our home and community and takes steps to eliminate them.

☐ We do a safety check of our home at least once a month, looking for ways to improve our safety.

☐ We store chemicals safely.

☐ Our family keeps stairs and high-traffic areas free of clutter.

☐ Family discussions remain calm and we look for compromises when conflicts arise.

☐ We talk about things that make us angry and explain our feelings calmly.

☐ We keep a list of emergency numbers near the telephone.

☐ Our fire safety plans include smoke detectors, fire extinguishers, and planned escape routes.

☐ We know and follow the safety rules for bicycling, swimming, and other outdoor activities.

☐ We keep a fully stocked first aid kit on hand to take care of minor injuries.

If you are interested in learning more about family safety, a good resource is:
***The Safe Child Book: A Commonsense Approach* (Fireside, 1996).**

Name: _____   Date: _____

INJURY PREVENTION

Write the word from the box that best completes each sentence.

hazard	chemical	unintentional
intersection		overload

1. A condition that creates a risk of danger is a _____.

2. Never cross the street against a light at an _____.

3. Mixing two cleaners could cause a _____ hazard.

4. Physical harm that is not deliberate is an _____ injury.

5. You should be careful not to _____ electrical outlets.

Write Safe or Not Safe for each statement. If not safe, write a related rule that is safe.

_____   6. Wrap tape around frayed or worn cords and plugs.

_____

_____   7. Always use a pot holder or a heat-resistant glove when handling items that have been in the oven.

_____

_____   8. Be very careful when hopping onto moving tractors or pick-up trucks.

_____

_____   9. If you see a hazard at school, report it to an adult.

_____

_____   10. Always get in or out of a car on the driver's side.

_____

Name: _____   Date: _____

INJURY PREVENTION

Match the words in Column A with the description in Column B.
Write the correct letter in the blank.

Column A

_____ **1.** unintentional injury

_____ **2.** overload

_____ **3.** intentional injury

_____ **4.** hazard

_____ **5.** thermostat

Column B

A. a condition or action that creates a risk of danger or physical harm

B. temperature control

C. deliberate physical harm to a person

D. physical harm that is not deliberate

E. plug too many appliances into one electrical outlet

Answer each question in complete sentences.

6. Can most unintentional injuries be avoided? Explain.

_____

7. What rule should you follow concerning electrical appliances and water?

_____

8. How can people get burned when no flame is visible?

_____

9. How can you make school fire drills effective?

_____

_____

10. What can you do to make your community a safer place?

_____

_____

McGraw-Hill School Division

Name: _____ Date: _____

VIOLENCE PREVENTION

Here are some sentences about violence prevention. Put a check mark in the blank beside each sentence that gives you good advice about how to avoid violence. Then explain why each sentence is or is not good advice. Use complete sentences.

_____ 1. Anger is a dangerous emotion, so you should never be angry.

_____

_____

_____ 2. Even though it can seem like a quick solution, violence is never a positive solution to any problem.

_____

_____

_____ 3. If someone acts violently toward you, you have no choice but to respond with violence.

_____

_____

_____ 4. One good way to resolve a conflict is to stay calm and allow each person the chance to explain his or her side.

_____

_____

_____

_____ 5. Compromises are only for situations that have already become violent.

_____

_____

_____

Name: _____   Date: _____

VIOLENCE PREVENTION

Complete the definition of each word.

1. Conflict is _____

2. Violence is _____

_____

3. To compromise is _____

4. A non-violent solution is_____

_____

5. Emotions are _____

Answer each question in complete sentences.

6. What can happen if feelings of anger are not dealt with properly?

_____

7. Why can't violence help to solve problems?

_____

8. Should you try to avoid all disagreements? Explain.

_____

_____

9. What can you do if you are angry with someone?

_____

10. If you are having a disagreement, is it better to use sentences that begin
    with "you or "I"? Explain.

_____

_____

Name: _____ Date: _____

INDOOR SAFETY

Underline the phrase that best completes each sentence.

1. A (sprain, bruise) is an injury to a part of your body that does not break the skin but causes it to change color.

2. A (sprain, bruise) is an injury caused by the sudden overstretching of a muscle.

3. To prevent falls and slips, you should wear (rubber-soled, dress shoes) when walking on slippery surfaces.

4. If you are home alone, you should never (let a stranger into your house, answer the phone).

5. If someone is poisoned, you should try to (throw the poison container away right away, save the poison container).

Write the word from the box that best completes each sentence.

```
stranger     never     poison

    always        emergency
```

6. You should _____ wipe up spilled liquids right away.

7. Never tell a _____ your name, address, or phone number.

8. A _____ is a substance that is harmful or deadly.

9. It's a good rule to keep a list of _____ phone numbers to use in case a problem arises.

10. To stay safe at home, _____ touch guns, even if you think they're not loaded.

Name: _____   Date: _____

INDOOR SAFETY

Write the word or phrase that best completes each sentence.

1. A situation that requires immediate help is an _____.

2. A substance that is harmful or deadly is a _____.

3. An injury to a part of the body that does not break the skin but breaks blood vessels, causing them to change color, is a _____.

4. An injury to a muscle or ligament caused by sudden overstretching is a _____.

5. You can help prevent slips and falls at home by using the _____ when you climb the stairs.

Answer each question in complete sentences.

6. What cleaning rules can help you prevent slips and falls at home?

    _____

7. Why is a local telephone book helpful in an emergency?

    _____

8. How should you answer the door if you are home alone?

    _____

    _____

9. Who should you call if someone accidentally swallows poison?

    _____

10. What information should you find out if someone has been poisoned?

    _____

    _____

McGraw-Hill School Division

Name: _____ Date: _____

FIRE SAFETY

Write the word or phrase from the box that best completes each sentence.

smoke	fire drill	flammable
fire extinguisher		smoke detector

1. There should be a _____ outside each sleeping area and at least one on every floor of a house.

2. You should never store _____ objects close to a radiator or fireplace.

3. The expiration date on a _____ tells you how long the chemicals are active.

4. If a room is filled with _____, cover your nose and mouth with a wet cloth and crawl low to the floor.

5. To help you plan your escape route in case of a fire, you can have a

    _____.

Write True or False for each statement. If false, change the underlined word or phrase to make it true.

_____ 6. Wood and plastic are common flammable materials.

_____ 7. Candles do not produce enough heat to be a hazard.

_____ 8. In case of a fire, you should try to fight the fire yourself.

_____ 9. You should activate a public fire alarm system as soon as you suspect a fire.

_____ 10. A good fire safety plan should include a meeting place outside the building.

Name: _____   Date: _____

FIRE SAFETY

Write the word or phrase that best completes each sentence.

1. A machine that sprays chemicals to put out a fire is a _____.

2. An item that is likely to catch fire easily and burn quickly is _____.

3. To make you aware of a fire because it sounds an alarm, you should have a _____.

4. What tells you how long the chemicals in a fire extinguisher last is the _____.

5. To help you plan an escape from a room or building in case of a fire, you should have a _____.

Answer each question in complete sentences.

6. How should flammable materials be stored?

   _____

   _____

7. How can space heaters be dangerous?

   _____

8. During a fire, why should you feel a door before opening it?

   _____

9. What should you do if your clothes catch fire?

   _____

10. What are the key features of a fire safety plan?

    _____

    _____

    _____

McGraw-Hill School Division

Name: _____   Date: _____

OUTDOOR SAFETY

Here are some sentences about outdoor safety. Put a check mark in the blank beside each sentence that gives you good advice about staying safe outdoors. Then explain why each sentence is or is not good advice. Use complete sentences.

_____ 1. If you are swimming at a lake, a good way to improve your endurance is to swim when you feel tired.

_____

_____

_____ 2. Everyone on a boat should wear a flotation device—even the good swimmers.

_____

_____

_____ 3. If someone is in trouble in the water, only a trained lifeguard should go into the water to try to rescue the swimmer.

_____

_____

_____ 4. The color of your clothing doesn't make any difference in hot and cold weather.

_____

_____

_____ 5. Traffic signs and lights are intended for cars, so bike riders don't need to follow the signs that seem confusing or inconvenient.

_____

_____

Name: _____ Date: _____

OUTDOOR SAFETY

Answer each question in complete sentences.

1. Frostbite is _____

_____

2. Heat exhaustion is _____

_____

3. Rescue breathing is _____

_____

4. Sunstroke is _____

_____

5. A personal flotation device is _____

_____

Write True or False for each statement. If false, change the underlined word or phrase to make it true.

_____ **6.** It is never safe to swim alone.

_____ **7.** If someone is in trouble in the water, anyone should try to rescue the person.

_____ **8.** To protect your skin from the sun, you can use sunscreen.

_____ **9.** For cold weather, dressing in layers will increase your heat loss.

_____ **10.** It is usually safe to wear headphones from a portable cassette player while you are bike riding.

Name: _____   Date: _____

EMERGENCIES AND FIRST AID

Underline the word or phrase that best completes each sentence.

1. People who are (unconscious, choking) are unaware of their surroundings.

2. An injury in which a bone is broken or cracked is a (puncture wound, fracture).

3. If a deep wound continues to bleed, you should (cover it with more bandages, remove the bandages).

4. In case of a fracture, you should use (bandages, ice) to reduce swelling.

5. To remove chemicals from a person's eyes, you should (rub vigorously with your hands, wash the eye gently with water).

6. (Paramedics, All adults) have special training in first aid and emergency medical procedures.

7. (Any trained person, Only a doctor) can help a person who is choking.

Read about each injury and tell how you would help.

8.

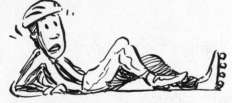

A boy sprains his ankle.   _____
_____
_____

9.

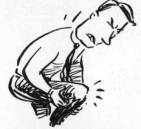

A man bruises his knee.   _____
_____
_____

10.

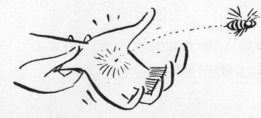

A girl gets stung by a bee.   _____
_____
_____

Name: _____   Date: _____

EMERGENCIES AND FIRST AID

Write the word or phrase that best completes each sentence.

1. A person who is trained to give first aid or emergency treatment is called a _____.

2. When a man is _____, he is unaware of his surroundings.

3. A type of injury in which a bone is broken or cracked is a _____.

4. A type of injury in which something pierces the skin, making a hole, is a _____.

5. When a woman is _____, her airway is blocked and she cannot breathe.

Answer each question in complete sentences.

6. How should you treat a minor cut or scrape?

_____

_____

7. What steps can you take to help a boy who has sprained his ankle?

_____

_____

8. What should you do in case of an emergency?

_____

_____

9. Should you wash a serious burn? Explain.

_____

10. How can you help a person who is unconscious while waiting for help to arrive?

_____

Name: _____ Date: _____

SAFETY, INJURY, AND VIOLENCE PREVENTION

Write the word or phrase from the box that best completes each sentence.

fracture	hazard	bruise	sunstroke	sprain
frostbite	unconscious	conflict	compromise	flammable

1. When people _____, they settle a disagreement.

2. A type of injury in which a bone is broken or cracked is a _____.

3. Intense cold can cause _____.

4. A muscle injury caused by overstretching is a _____.

5. An injury to a part of the body that does not break the skin but causes it to change color is a _____.

6. Staying too long in the sun can cause _____.

7. Something that is _____ is likely to catch fire easily.

8. A disagreement between two or more people creates _____.

9. A condition that creates a risk of danger is a _____.

10. A person who is unaware of his surroundings is _____.

Circle the letter of the best answer.

11. Using violence to solve a problem is
    a. a compromise   **b.** never successful   **c.** sometimes unavoidable

12. Flammable materials should be stored
    a. inside heat sources   **b.** next to heat sources   **c.** away from heat sources

13. When home alone, you should never
    a. make phone calls   **b.** call for help   **c.** let a stranger inside

Name: _____   Date: _____

SAFETY, INJURY, AND VIOLENCE PREVENTION

14. One smart rule to follow when bike riding is to

    a. wear a helmet   **b.** wear headphones   **c.** wear dark clothing

15. To help an unconscious person before paramedics arrive, you should

    a. raise the legs   **b.** cover the person   **c.** use ice packs
                          with a blanket

Answer each question in complete sentences.

16. What is the difference between an intentional and an unintentional injury?

_____

_____

17. One of your friends is involved in a very angry discussion. How can you help prevent the situation from turning violent?

_____

_____

_____

18. What can you do to help when someone is poisoned?

_____

_____

19. What should you do if you are on land and you see a swimmer having trouble in the water?

_____

_____

20. How can you help a person who has a minor burn?

_____

Extra Credit: On a separate sheet of paper, describe one common source of home injuries. Give three safety rules that help you and your family avoid this type of injury.

Name: _____   Date: _____

Dear Parent or Guardian,

We are about to start **Chapter 10, Community and Environmental Health**, in which we will explore this Big Idea:

> Various groups and individuals in your community provide health care for you and your family and promote the health of your environment.

Your child will be learning about

- the people and facilities that make up the community health care system

- how public health laws and services protect you and your community and provide help in times of crisis

- how air and noise pollution can affect your health

- the effects of land and water pollution and how to control them

Help your child fill out the checklist below. Talk about how practicing ideas from the checklist can help your family recognize the importance of community and environmental health.

Community and Environmental Health
Family Checklist

☐ Our family is familiar with the different kinds of health care workers and services in our community.

☐ We are aware that some claims about what a medical service or product can do are false, and ask health care workers for guidance.

☐ We know there are public laws that protect our health and public services to help in times of need.

☐ We help our community by following sanitation regulations.

☐ We know that loud noises and air pollution can damage our health.

☐ We are aware of how our community tries to protect our land and water.

☐ All family members help control pollution and waste by conserving natural resources; reducing, reusing, and recycling; and by spreading the word about pollution.

If you are interested in learning more about community and environmental health, some good resources are: *The Consumer Health Information Source Book*, (Oryx Press, 1994), and *The Kid's Guide to Service Projects* (Free Spirit, 1995).

Grade 5, Chapter 10

Name: _____ Date: _____

COMMUNITY HEALTH CARE

Write the word or phrase from the box that best completes each sentence.

| clinic | hospice | nurse | paramedic | pediatrician |
| pharmacist | physical therapist | physician assistant |

1. A person who prepares medicines according to a doctor's orders is a
   _____ .

2. A doctor who takes care of babies is a _____ .

3. In a _____ you get medical treatment at little cost.

4. A person who might perform a medical procedure on you, under your doctor's supervision, is a _____ .

5. You might work with a _____ if you injure a leg or other part of your body and need help recovering.

6. A person who is very ill or dying might go to a _____ .

7. In a medical emergency, a _____ might assist a person in an ambulance on the way to a hospital.

8. If you're sick or injured, the person who might take care of you or assist your doctor is a _____ .

Answer each question in complete sentences.

9. What is the purpose of a community immunization program?

   _____

   _____

10. What is the difference between an inpatient and an outpatient?

    _____

Name: _____   Date: _____

COMMUNITY HEALTH CARE

Match the word or phrase in Column A with the description in Column B.
Write the correct letter in the column.

Column A

_____ **1.** certified

_____ **2.** clinic

_____ **3.** health care delivery system

_____ **4.** public health system

_____ **5.** quackery

Column B

A. the selling of medical products and services that make false claims

B. a health care facility where patients can be treated, often at little or no cost

C. network of government departments that provide health education, disease control, and a clean environment

D. officially approved or licensed to provide a service

E. people who provide medical services

Answer each question in complete sentences.

6. In what ways do your state and local health departments protect your health?

_____

_____

7. What are two examples of quackery?

_____

8. In case of illness or injury, why should you call your family doctor first?

_____

9. How does the licensing of health care workers protect your health?

_____

10. What should you do before you use any health-related product you see advertised on TV or in a magazine?

_____

Name: _____   Date: _____

PUBLIC HEALTH LAWS AND SERVICES

Complete each sentence with a word or phrase that makes the sentence true.

1. Garbage collection is one aspect of public _____ that is regulated in most communities.

2. Health department inspectors check restaurants and food stores to make sure the owners are following _____.

3. To protect your heath, your drinking water is checked for _____.

4. Many communities have laws that forbid _____ in public places to protect people from the harmful effects of passive smoke.

5. In a crisis, such as an earthquake or a _____, the government or private groups may offer disaster relief.

6. You can look in the phonebook to find a _____ number to call in a crisis.

Write True or False for each statement. If the statement is false, change the underlined word or phrase to make it true.

_____   7. One way to help keep your community underline{messy} is by recycling.

_____   8. Another way to help keep your community healthy is by underline{using} household products that contain harmful chemicals.

_____   9. To ask for help in an emergency, a underline{community hot line} is a good place to call.

_____   10. Disaster underline{relief} is the support that is given to people in time of crises.

Name: _____   Date: _____

PUBLIC HEALTH LAWS AND SERVICES

Write the word or phrase from the box that best competes each sentence.

disaster relief   hot line   sanitation   voluntary health agency

1. A phone number to call in an emergency is a _____.

2. A group of people who donate their time and effort to work for community health needs is a _____.

3. Help provided to people in times of disaster is _____.

4. The maintenance of a clean and healthful environment is _____.

Answer each question in complete sentences.

5. Why do governments pass rules and regulations against pollution?

_____

6. How does placing trash in tightly covered containers help keep your community healthy?

_____

7. How do community health care services aid in disease prevention and control?

_____

_____

8. What kinds of services might disaster relief consist of?

_____

9. How do voluntary health agencies offer support in times of crisis?

_____

10. What is a voluntary health agency?

_____

_____

Name: _____ Date: _____

AIR AND NOISE POLLUTION

Write the word or phrase from the box that best completes each sentence.

| asbestos   carbon monoxide   lead   smog   soot |

1. A substance found in exhaust from vehicles that causes damage to the nervous system is _____.

2. A pollutant produced by wood-burning stoves and exhaust from some factories is _____.

3. A combination of smoke, fog, and exhaust that you may not be able to see is _____.

4. Insulation in some buildings contains _____, which scars lungs and can cause cancer.

5. An air pollutant that reduces the oxygen level in the blood is _____.

Underline the phrase that best completes each sentence.

6. In emphysema, the (alveoli, tumors) of the lungs are damaged, making it difficult to take in oxygen.

7. The ozone layer protects the earth from (harmful rays from the sun, exhaust from wood-burning stoves).

8. Long-term exposure to loud noise can damage the (bronchial tubes, nerve cells) in your ears.

9. The higher the decibel level, the (louder, softer) the sound.

10. Living in a noisy environment can (lower your ability to concentrate, raise the level of smog in your community).

McGraw-Hill School Division

Name: _____   Date: _____

AIR AND NOISE POLLUTION

Use a word or phrase to complete each definition.

1. A disease in which uncontrollable cell growth causes tumors that destroy the lungs is _____.

2. A lung disease in which the linings of tubes connecting the windpipe to the lungs become inflamed is _____.

3. An unhealthful substance that makes the air, water, or soil dirty or impure is a _____.

4. A lung disease in which air passages become narrow, making breathing difficult is _____.

5. A disease which affects the alveoli, making it difficult for the body to take in oxygen is _____.

Answer each question in complete sentences.

6. What steps can people take to protect themselves during a smog alert?

   _____

   _____

7. Why is soot considered harmful to your health?

   _____

8. What are some common sources of noise pollution?

   _____

9. What can you do to help control noise pollution?

   _____

   _____

10. What are some sources of air pollution?

   _____

Name: _____ Date: _____

LAND AND WATER POLLUTION

Identify the source of water or land pollution shown in each picture.

1.
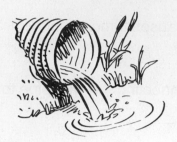
_____

2.
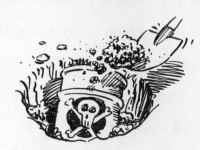
_____

3.
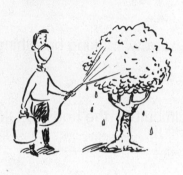
_____

4.
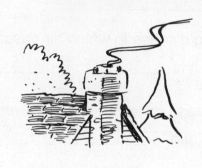
_____

Underline the word or phrase that best completes each sentence.

5. To reduce the threat of toxic wastes, wastes are dumped and buried in (groundwater, a landfill).

6. One way to dispose of wastes is to burn them in (an incinerator, a recycling center).

7. In a water treatment plant, (a pesticide, chlorine) is used to kill bacteria.

8. When you don't buy products with unnecessary packaging, you are (reusing, reducing) wastes.

9. Two natural resources are (water and forests, acids and plastics).

10. To spread the word about pollution to other people, suggest that they (throw away all glass and metal items, find other uses for discarded items).

Name: _____ Date: _____

LAND AND WATER POLLUTION

Match the word or phrase in Column A with the description in Column B.
Write the correct letter in the blank.

Column A	Column B
_____ 1. acid rain	**A.** waste water from buildings
_____ 2. pesticide	**B.** the process of cleaning or removing poisons from something
_____ 3. purification	**C.** a chemical used to kill insects
_____ 4. sewage	**D.** trash or waste material that contains poisonous substances
_____ 5. toxic waste	**E.** chemicals that mix with moisture in the air and fall back to earth

Answer each question in complete sentences.

6. In what ways can you become ill from polluted water?

_____

7. What can happen if groundwater gets polluted?

_____

8. How does hot water from factories pollute waterways?

_____

_____

9. How does using energy-efficient appliances help control pollution?

_____

10. How is recycling different from reusing?

_____

_____

Name: _____   Date: _____

COMMUNITY AND ENVIRONMENTAL HEALTH

Write the word or phrase from the box that best completes each sentence.

bronchitis	clinic	quackery	certified	disaster relief
toxic waste	asthma	purification	hot line	sanitation

1. A lung disease in which air passages become narrow, making breathing difficult, is _____.

2. Trash or waste that contains poisonous substances is _____.

3. The maintenance of a clean and healthful environment is _____.

4. A lung disease in which the linings of tubes connecting the windpipe to the lungs become inflamed is _____.

5. To be licensed to provide a service is to be _____.

6. The process of cleaning or removing poisons is _____.

7. A number that people call in an emergency is a _____.

8. A facility where patients are treated at little cost is a _____.

9. Help provided to people by government or private groups in times of disaster, such as a flood or an earthquake, is _____.

10. The selling of products that make false claims is _____.

Write True or False for each statement. If false, change the underlined word or phrase to make it true.

_____ 11. You might need the help of a voluntary health organization as a result of a <u>tornado</u>.

_____ 12. Water between rocks and soil beneath the earth's surface forms <u>the ozone layer</u>.

Name: _____   Date: _____

COMMUNITY AND ENVIRONMENTAL HEALTH

_____   **13.** When you need a toothache treated, you would go to a <u>dentist</u>.

_____   **14.** A decibel is a unit that measures the <u>degree of air pollution</u>.

Answer each question in complete sentences.

15. Why is it important to know about pollutants?

_____

16. What is the purpose of a sewage treatment plant?

_____

17. What does a state or local health department usually keep records of?

_____

18. How can agencies like the American Diabetes Association and the American Heart Association help people?

_____

19. What kind of promises might an ad make that would lead you to believe it's an example of quackery?

_____

20. What is one source of land pollution that could directly affect your health, and how could you protect yourself from it?

_____

_____

Extra Credit: On a separate piece of paper, write a paragraph describing how you could promote the health of your community or environment.

McGraw-Hill School Division